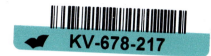

Aspects of Modern Otolaryngological Practice

Advances in
Oto-Rhino-Laryngology

Vol. 29

Series Editor
C. R. Pfaltz, Basel

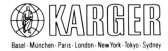

Basel · München · Paris · London · New York · Tokyo · Sydney

Aspects of Modern Otolaryngological Practice

Volume Editors
S. Prasansuk, Bangkok
C. Bunnag, Bangkok
P. Srisomboon, Bangkok

149 figures and 49 tables, 1983

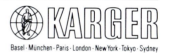

KARGER

Basel · München · Paris · London · New York · Tokyo · Sydney

Advances in Oto-Rhino-Laryngology

Drug Dosage

The author and publisher have exerted every effort to ensure that drug selection and dosage set forth in this text are in accord with current recommendations and practice at the time of publication. However, in view of ongoing research, changes in government regulations, and the constant flow of information relating to drug therapy and drug reactions, the reader is urged to check the package insert for each drug for any change in indications and dosage and for added warnings and precautions. This is particularly important when the recommended agent is a new and/or infrequently employed drug.

Contents

Contents

The ASEAN Otorhinolaryngological Federation

Committee Members 1980–1981

President	Purnaman S. Pandi, MD, FICS
	Jarkarta, Indonesia
Vice-President	Mariano B. Caparas, MD
	Manila, Philippines
Secretary General and Treasurer	Suchitra Prasansuk MD, DLO, FICS
	Bangkok, Thailand
Committee Members	U. Prasad, MD
	Kuala Lumpur, Malaysia
	N. Kunaratnam, MD
	Singapore

Committee Members 1982–1983

President	Prasit Srisomboon, MD, FICS, FACS
	Bangkok, Thailand
Vice-President	A. Gnanapragasam, MBBS, FRCS, DLO, FICS,
	Kuala Lumpur, Malaysia
Secretary General and Treasurer	Suchitra Prasansuk, MD, DLO, FICS
	Bangkok, Thailand
Committee Members	Mariano B. Caparas, MD
	Manila, Philippines
	Purnaman S. Pandi, MD, FICS
	Jarkarta, Indonesia
	N. Kunaratnam
	Singapore

Office: Department of Otolaryngology, Faculty of Medicine and Siriraj Hospital, Mahidol University, Bangkok 10700, Thailand.
Tel.: 411-4816, 411-3254

The First ASEAN ORL Congress

Organizing Committee

Honourary President	Chern Sekorarith, MD, FICS, FACS Associate Professor in Otolaryngology Department of Otolaryngology Faculty of Medicine and Siriraj Hospital Mahidol University, Bangkok
President	Prasit Srisomboon, MD, FICS, FACS Assistant Professor in Otolaryngology Department of Otolaryngology Faculty of Medicine and Siriraj Hospital Mahidol University, Bangkok
Secretary General and Treasurer	Suchitra Prasansuk, MD, DLO, FICS Associate Professor in Otolaryngology Department of Otolaryngology Faculty of Medicine and Siriraj Hospital Mahidol University, Bangkok
Chairman Scientific Programme Organization	Chaweewan Bunnag, MD, FICS Associate Professor in Otolaryngology Department of Otolaryngology Faculty of Medicine and Siriraj Hospital Mahidol University, Bangkok
Technical Exhibition	Prathan Sutaputa, MD, FACS Samithivej Hospital, Bangkok
Social Programme	Poonpit Amatyakul, MD, MS Audiology Associate Professor in Otolaryngology Faculty of Medicine, Ramathibodi Hospital Bangkok
Public Relations and Information	Salyaveth Lekagul, MD, FACS Department of Otolaryngology Faculty of Medicine, Chulalongkorn Hospital Bangkok

Committee Members

Major General Aswin Debhakam
Pramongkut Krao Medical College
Bangkok

Chira Siribodhi
Hua Cheo Hospital
Bangkok

Choo Chuang Sevetarundra
Associate Professor in Otolaryngology
Department of Otolaryngology
Faculty of Medicine, Chulalongkorn Hospital
Bangkok

Kob-Kiat Ruckphaopunt
Associate Professor in Otolaryngology
Department of Otolaryngology
Faculty of Medicine, Chieng Mai University
Chieng Mai

Kosol Lekhavat
Associate Professor in Otolaryngology
Department of Otolaryngology
Faculty of Medicine, Chulalongkorn Hospital
Bangkok

Prapote Clongsusuek
Associate Professor in Otolaryngology
Department of Otolaryngology
Faculty of Medicine, Ramathibodi Hospital
Bangkok

Col. Serm Rusakul
Pramongkut Krao Medical College
Bangkok

Soontorn Antarasena
Rajvithi Hospital
Bangkok

Susawat Saihoo
Assistant Professor in Otolaryngology
Department of Otolaryngology
Faculty of Medicine and Siriraj Hospital
Mahidol University
Bangkok

Preface

There are a number of problems which are common to the peoples of South-East Asia. It was therefore not surprising that, in August 1967, the foreign ministers of Indonesia, Malaysia, the Philippines, Singapore and Thailand agreed to form a non-military association for political cooperation. This association is termed the Association of South-East Asian Nations (ASEAN).

Subsequent events have shown that the meaning which the ASEAN peoples have attached to the term 'politics' in this context has been all-embracing. Indeed, in the words of Gouverneur *Morris,* who was a delegate at the convention which framed the United States Constitution in 1787, politics is that 'sublime science which embraces for its object the happiness of mankind'.

It was therefore natural that organizations concerned with health care should spring up under the ASEAN umbrella. In particular, the Federation of the ASEAN Otolaryngological Society was founded in Medan, Indonesia, on July 2, 1980.

At the meeting in Medan, it was agreed that the ASEAN Otolaryngological Federation should promote congresses wherein mutual otolaryngologic problems could be discussed and new relevant knowledge in the field highlighted. With this in mind, the Otolaryngological Society of Thailand in cooperation with the Department of Otolaryngology, Siriraj Hospital, Mahidol University, Bangkok, agreed to organize the First Congress of the Federation. This took place in Pattaya, Thailand, in December 1981.

The Organizing Committee were unanimous that, since ASEAN otolaryngologists were anxious to hear about new developments which could have a bearing on their own practice, it would be most appropriate to include speakers from outside the region. Indeed, the Organizing Committee were fortunate in recruiting 26 guest speakers who represented 10 countries outside the ASEAN grouping. Moreover, this has meant that the organizing committee were able to tap the expertise of all five continents. Thus, what could initially be claimed to be an international meeting became a world event.

The Organizing Committee were so impressed with the standard and variety of these invited papers that they have arranged for their publication. The contents of this book should be of interest not only to the otolaryngologist of South-East Asia, but also to all those throughout the world.

S. Prasansuk, Bangkok

Adv. Oto-Rhino-Laryng., vol. 29, pp. 1–5 (Karger, Basel 1983)

The History of Otorhinolaryngology in Thailand

Porn Varavej

Previous Chief, Department of Otolaryngology,
Siriraj Hospital, Mahidol University, Bangkok, Thailand

I am greatly honored to be invited by the organizing committee to give a summary of the history of the development of otorhinolaryngology in Thailand.

I know that many of you have travelled long distances to attend this international meeting, and as a senior member of this association, I would like to bid you all a hearty welcome. Although we may live in different parts of the world, speak different languages, believe in different religions and possess diverse cultures, I am sure we shall become good friends at this meeting. We shall share our knowledge, exchange ideas and learn from each other with the ultimate goal of relieving the suffering of patients with ear, nose, throat and larynx diseases. In the past we have made significant contributions towards lessening human distress and in future we shall continue with the same aim.

The history of otorhinolaryngology in Thailand dates back many decades to the years of World War I – 1914–1918. In this war we joined the allies and in 1918 a token force was sent to fight in France. Three Thai doctors accompanied this small force and saw action in the last battles of the war. When the war ended, these 3 doctors, *Luang Baed Kosol, Luang Kosol Veshasatra* and *Luang Prachack,* were permitted by the army to attend postgraduate courses in England; the first two were interested in otolaryngology and the third one specialized in ophthalmology. The former two returned home and became staff at the Chulalongkorn Red Cross Hospital. They were the nucleus of the future department and played an important role in the advances of otolaryngology. Besides working at Chulalongkorn Hospital they also had private clinics. Although I am not familiar personally with these two doctors and have no details of their work and accomplishments, their names are well known not only in the medical circle but also in philanthropy. In the latter part of their lives they gave generous support to the medical school and religious organizations. Undoubtedly we can be proud of our predecessors in otolaryngology, both made valuable contributions for the benefit of the people of the country.

When we talk about the history of otolaryngology we cannot omit the history of medical education, both are involved in the development of each other. The year 1900 saw the establishment of our first medical school with a curriculum of 5 years and this was lengthened to 6 years when the Rockefeller Foundation first gave assistance to our medical school in 1922. Besides laying a modern basis to our curriculum the Rockefeller Foundation also gave scholarships for our doctors to further their studies in the United States and other countries, and also recruited distinguished physicians and surgeons to teach at our medical school. During my premedical years I can well remember attending lectures in nearly every subject with teachers from many countries. At that time, Prof. *Thomas Paterson Noble* was the head of the Department of Surgery and it can be said that he was the father of general surgery and also otolaryngology in Thailand.

Prof. *Noble* had a distinguished career, he was a Fellow of the Royal College of Surgeons of London and also Fellow of the Royal Society of Edinburgh. He served in World War I for many years with the British army. When the war ended he became a orthopedic surgeon at the Mayo Clinic, USA. In 1926 he was selected by the Rockefeller Foundation as the chief of the Department of Surgery of our Siriraj Medical School, at the same time he also made plans to establish an otorhinolaryngology department.

In 1928 one of the staff of the Department of Surgery, Dr. *Daeng Kanchanaran*, obtained a scholarship from the Rockefeller Foundation for 2 years postgraduate study in ophthalmology and otolaryngology in India. On his return, Dr. *Daeng* became chief of the eye, ear, nose and throat section in the Department of Surgery. Dr. *Daeng*, or Prof. Dr. *Daeng Kanchanaran*, made a great name in our speciality during his time.

In my final year as a medical student in 1934 I was very interested in the subject of eye, ear, nose and throat and at the end of my medical school years, I applied to work in this section and was accepted as the first resident. I was elected to be a permanent staff member in the following year.

In the early years the eye, ear, nose and throat section was part of the Department of Surgery. In the outpatient department we had a small table, working side by side with the general surgeons. Our admissions were into the same wards and the operations were scheduled in the same two existing rooms at that time. However, being a new and junior unit we had to operate very early in the morning and be out of the operating rooms by 9 a.m. when our big brothers the general surgeons and gynecologists would take over. The routine operations in the early years consisted of basic cataract extraction, tonsillectomy, polypectomy, etc. Tonsillectomy was first operated by Dr. *Daeng* using the guillotine method and later I was trained to the dissection technique by Prof. *Noble* – also, it was the rule that every tonsillectomy operation had to have a final approval for 'no bleeding' by Prof. *Noble*.

In 1940 we expanded our department and recruited more staff members and my own work increased towards otolaryngology more than ophthalmology, although we were still combined in the same department. At that time, the use of prophylactic diphtheria immunization was not widely employed and we had many cases of children and infants in which emergency tracheotomy had to be performed in the middle of the night. I was also responsible for cases of foreign bodies in the pharynx, esophagus, trachea and bronchus. Although we had a complete set of Chavelier-Jackson's laryngobronchoesophagoscopy instruments, no one was familiar with the technique of using it. We were helpless and could only watch many deaths from complications of false teeth, fish and chicken bones impacted in the esophagus. Later we obtained a textbook of otorhinolaryngology by *Jackson and Jackson,* and began to learn the technique from this book. However, it took some years before instrumentation could be performed with any degree of confidence and competence. This shows that learning surgery by textbook without good teachers is a very slow process.

I remember one early case in 1948. I had a male Thai patient of 60 years of age who ate a potato-like vegetable which became inpacted at the cardiac end of the esophagus. He could neither eat nor drink. Finally he reluctantly allowed me to use the esophagoscope, but this vegetable was very brittle and every time I attempted to remove it with forceps it would break into small pieces. After about 10 minutes the patient refused to tolerate any further manipulations because of pressure of the instrument on his gum caused considerable pain. As this was one of my first esophagoscopies it was not surprising that I could not remove the foreign body but the patient immediately sat up, smiled dryly and said that he felt much better with no more obstruction and could now drink water. This was one dramatic but doubtful success in the fight against impacted foreign bodies. Later I presented a paper on '10 cases of foreign bodies in the esophagus' at the faculty meeting and published it in the *Journal of the Medical Association of Thailand* in 1948. Many other papers on foreign bodies followed this first publication.

At the end of World War II, I received funds from ICA to spend a year as a fellow at Barnes Hospital, St. Louis, Mo., working in the ear, nose, and throat department with Prof. *Walse* and Prof. *Ogura*. It was a most useful and enjoyable year and I learned a great deal from these two kind teachers. On returning home, newer operations such as rhinoplasty, radical mastoidectomy, arytenoidectomy and others were developed rapidly.

Although some advances were made in otolaryngology it was generally felt that progress was slow as we were still grouped in the same department as general surgery. In 1945, ophthalmology and otolaryngology was officially set up as a new department separate from general surgery. Although we had our own wards for admission of patients, we still utilized the same operating rooms. My work at this time consisted mostly of otolaryngology and I felt that the next step would be to separate ophthalmology and otolaryngology into two departments as practised in most hospitals. To prepare for this separation when Prof. *Daeng* retired and I was elected in his place, the staff were requested to divide themselves unofficially into sections of ophthalmology and otolaryngology and work in separate fields. It was not until 1970 that ophthalmology and otolaryngology were officially separated and I became the head of the new otolaryngology department. This was the realization of my dream after 30 years hard work, but many problems still remained to be solved.

I feel most happy to report that the present staff have been well trained in many countries of the world. They are all working hard to bring progress to the Department. Now I believe that our Department is one of the best in this part of the world. It is well equipped both in the diagnostic clinics and in the operating rooms. Although my hope for an excellent department was not fully realized when I was chief of the Department many years ago, I feel justly proud, when I was recently conducted by my successor to see every nook and every corner of the Department. The success of the Department has given me great happiness in my declining years.

I have been recounting to you the history of the Otorhinolaryngology Department of Siriraj Hospital Medical School and it can be said that the Department played the part of the elder brother to the similar Departments in other medical schools and hospitals throughout the country. The reason for this is that the Siriraj Hospital Medical School was the first medical school of the country and remained the only one for nearly 50 years. Thus, the graduates from Siriraj migrated into the towns and villages wherever medicine is practised. Many send patients or write letters for consultation with the result that for many years we were flooded with otolaryngologic patients, giving us a great deal of material for our experiences, for training our residents and for any research projects. Now trained staff in otolaryngology can be found in the large hospitals of Bangkok and the large cities.

With the rapid increase in population it was necessary to graduate more doctors, and this situation was made worse by the 'brain drain' to the USA. With this in mind the authorities of Siriraj Hospital Medical School established a new medical school at Chulalongkorn Red Cross Hospital in 1959, and later other medical schools were created in the North, North-East and Southern regions of the country. The latest one is the Armed Forces Medical School in Bangkok. This then is the summary of the history of otorhinolaryngology in this country as far as my memory has served me.

Prof. Porn Varavej, Previous Chief, Department of Otolaryngology, Siriraj Hospital, Mahidol University, Bangkok 7 (Thailand)

Adv. Oto-Rhino-Laryng., vol. 29, pp. 6–8 (Karger, Basel 1983)

Some Thoughts on the Current Management of Laryngeal Cancer

D.F.N. Harrison

Institute of Laryngology and Otology, University of London, London, England

The mortality for laryngeal cancer in England and Wales between 1911 and 1978 shows an increase for men of 28/million in 1911 to a peak of 60/million in the 1930s. The age-adjusted mortality rate in 1978 was 25/million. This decline occurred at a period of reduced alcohol consumption but an increase in cigarette smoking. However, in females the rates for both laryngeal and bronchial cancer are rising rapidly. Almost certainly this is due to the increase in smoking amongst women since World War II. Standardized registration ratios for laryngeal cancer in women were 87 in 1966 and in 1978 had risen to 165. The increased rates in city dwellers as opposed to urban communities in both bronchial and laryngeal cancer sufferers is probably attributed more to differences in smoking habits rather than air pollution.

There are wide variations in the incidence of laryngeal cancer between various countries. Japan has about 30/million in men – 150/million in parts of Spain – and in the UK an incidence of about 55/million in men. Variations in incidence rates are found between different parts of most countries and the epidemiologist is now accepted as a vital part of the investigatory team.

In the early part of this century most cases of laryngeal cancer were treated by surgery with the first total laryngectomy being carried out in 1873. Around 1920 radiotherapy began to be accepted as a worthwhile form of therapy and the surgical pendulum did not swing again until the 1950s with the introduction of conservation surgical techniques.

Poor radiotherapy is undoubtedly worse for the patient than poor surgery and the more acceptable combinations of primary curative doses of radiotherapy followed by salvage surgery are dependent upon the availability of skilled radiotherapists with modern, accurately calibrated equipment.

The risk of recurrence or residual disease is largely related to the initial extent of the tumour as well as its histological differentiation. A figure of 15% for primary glottic to almost 100% for transglottic neoplasms would be realistic.

Unfortunately, as will be discussed in my second lecture, the intrinsic errors in the existing TNM system of classification makes interpretation of most of the larger published series involving treatment of laryngeal cancer, debatable. In countries possessing effective departments of radiotherapy, and appreciating the considerable socio-economic disabilities secondary to total laryngectomy, most laryngeal cancers are treated primarily with radiotherapy. Total laryngectomy is then used for patients with residual disease or local recurrence although in the 15% of uncontrolled glottic tumours – vertical partial laryngectomy (laryngofissure approach) will salvage at least half of these patients. Horizontal supraglottic laryngectomy is less favoured since many think the long-term results are little better than with curative doses of radiotherapy and case selection demands considerable experience. In the more advanced tumours with cord fixation or possible cartilage invasion primary radiotherapy by producing surface healing and oedema of arytenoids and aryepiglottic folds, frequently masks deeply placed residual cancer. T_3 and T_4 tumours may therefore be better treated by a combination of 4,000 rad cobalt followed by total laryngectomy. Once again, the relative effectiveness of these various regimes are difficult to evaluate due to classification errors.

If a patient is undergoing total or partial laryngectomy and has regional lymph node metastases then a concomitant radical neck dissection is necessary. Curative dose radiotherapy to high risk neck nodes in the clinically negative neck has now replaced 'prophylactic' neck dissection. Whether a 'conservation' neck dissection has anything worth while to offer in the management of laryngeal cancer has yet to be established. Little is known of the social and economic consequences of total laryngectomy in the various ethnic groups and countries of the world. This is an effective oncological operation with good prospects of long life and even adequate powers of communication. Oesophageal voice, whether self-taught or professionally taught, can be obtained in at least 50% of men and the more recent tracheal-oesophageal shunts may yet play an important role in the voice failures.

However, the effect of laryngeal loss on work capabilities and family relationships is largely unexplored and may well influence initial choice of therapy. This is a rich field of research in the Asian countries and requires not finance but concern.

D.F.N. Harrison, MD, Institute of Laryngology and Otology,
University of London, 330 Gray's Inn Road, London WC 1 (England)

Adv. Oto-Rhino-Laryng., vol. 29, pp. 9–23 (Karger, Basel 1983)

Growth and Spread of Laryngeal Cancer[1]

Douglas P. Bryce[a], *A.W. Peter van Nostrand*[b], *Ivan Brodarec*[c]

Departments of [a] Otolaryngology and [b] Pathology, University of Toronto, Toronto General Hospital, Toronto, Canada; [c] Department of Otolaryngology, University of Zagreb, University Hospital 'Dr. M. Stojanovic', Zagreb, Yugoslavia

Applied Anatomy

There are several fundamentally important features of laryngeal anatomy which profoundly affect the spread of tumours within the larynx and which also dictate and influence the design of the surgical approaches to the irradication of laryngeal malignancy.

Embryologically, the supraglottis is distinct from the glottis and also differs in that the glottis develops as a paired structure while the supraglottis does not. Thus, tumours are reluctant to invade the glottis from the supraglottis and spread from one side of the glottis to the other. Circumferential spread in the supra- and subglottis is not restricted.

The anatomical features of the anterior commissure, the conus elasticus and posterior commissure influence the direction and extent of tumour spread as does the pattern of blood supply in the glottis and the distribution of mucous glands in the glottis and the subglottis.

As seen in figure 1, at the anterior commissure, the fibrous structure of the vocal cords melds into the perichondrium and thus presents an avascular, very strong barrier to spread of tumour from one cord to the other. There is no depth to the glottis at this point, whereas in the mid-cord region the vocal cord has a depth of 4—5 mm (fig. 2). The conus elasticus forms the mobile portion of the laryngeal subglottic (fig. 3). As such, it acts as an effective barrier for tumour spread from the glottis to the subglottis. The conus is a very strong fibrous structure (fig. 4). The mobile subglottis is about 1 cm in depth anteriorly, but this depth disappears at the posterior commissure (fig. 5).

The vasculature in the glottis flows anteriorly and posteriorly

---

[1] This work was supported by the Charlie Conacher Cancer Research Fund.

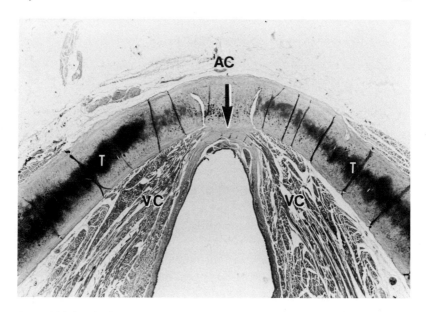

Fig. 1. This is a horizontal section at the level of the vocal cord to demonstrate the anatomy of the anterior commissure (AC). A blending of the fibrous structure of the vocal cord (VC) is illustrated which melds into the perichondrium of the thyroid alae (T).

(fig. 6) and the pattern of tumour spread on the vocal cord follows this pathway. There are no mucous glands in the mucosa of the vocal cord, but they appear immediately in the subglottis and may assist in the circumferential spread of tumour in this area.

In the supraglottis, the commonest site of tumour is the infrahyoid epiglottis where the tumour tends to remain confined for some time (fig. 7 a—c). The pre-epiglottic space is an anatomical feature of great importance as tumours in this space may extend from side to side without barrier of any kind (fig. 8). It is extremely important to realize also that the tumour in the pre-epiglottic space may be beneath the vallecula and invade the base of the tongue without such spread being in evidence clinically.

Spread of Glottic Tumours (table I)

The commonest site of origin for glottic tumours is the anterior third of one vocal cord. Tumours here are remarkably localized (fig. 9)

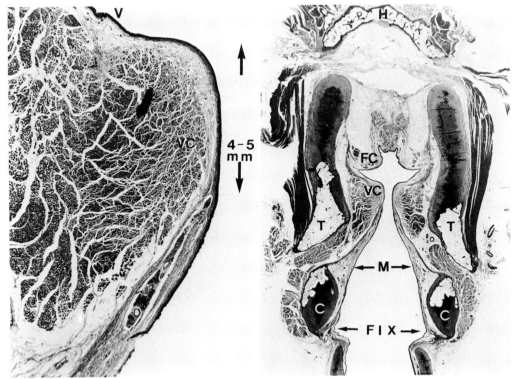

2   3

Fig. 2. Coronal section of the anterior portion of a vocal cord (VC) demonstrating its depth and its muscular and epithelial structure. The absence of glands at the free edges of the true vocal cord is noted, but their reappearance in the immediate subglottic area, external to the conus elasticus, is demonstrated. The free margin of the true cord is limited to 4–5 mm in vertical extent. V = Laryngeal ventricle.

Fig. 3. Coronal section of the larynx in its anterior third clearly demonstrating the anatomical features. The dominant feature of the conus elasticus separating the glottis from the subglottis is well demonstrated in this section. H = Hyoid bone; FC = false cord; VC = vocal cord; T = thyroid; M = mobile subglottis; FIX = fixed subglottis; C = cricoid cartilage.

and are highly curable. As the tumour grows, it spreads anteriorly and posteriorly along the cord and it reaches the anterior commissure where the conus elasticus and anterior commissure tendon strongly resist its further growth (fig. 10, 11). The musculature of the cord is then involved (fig. 12) and at the same time, the ventricle may be crossed. Invasion of the subglottis results from destruction of the conus elasticus, so that tumour spreading from one side to the other at the commis-

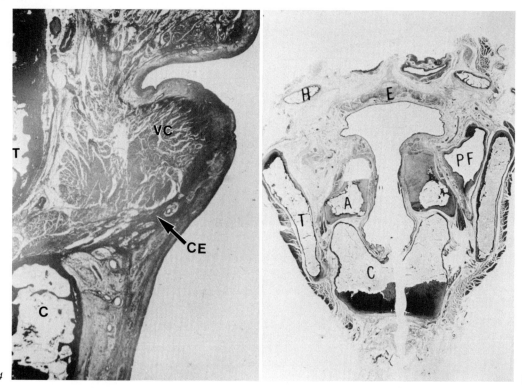

4
5

Fig. 4. High-power view of the vocal cord and immediate subglottis demonstrating by elastic stain the very strong conus elasticus (CE) which acts as a formidable barrier for the spread of malignant disease from the glottis to the subglottis. T = Thyroid cartilage; VC = vocal cord; C = cricoid cartilage.

Fig. 5. This posterior coronal section of the larynx at the level of the arytenoid (A) and cricoid (C) articulation demonstrates the absence of the vertical depth of the mobile subglottis, posterior in the larynx. H = Hyoid bone; E = epiglottis; T = thyroid cartilage; PF = pyriform sinus.

sure are usually invasive and are extensive tumours. Extensive musculature involvement by tumour is the cause of cord fixation which is recognized clinically as a poor prognostic sign. Spread to the posterior commissure is usually late and here the tumour is no longer confined but may easily become subglottic or spread to the post-cricoid mucosa, either medially or laterally to the arytenoid which may be destroyed by tumour invasion (fig. 13, 14).

The routes of exit from the larynx of extensive tumour of the glottis are of great importance for the surgeon when a laryngectomy is to be

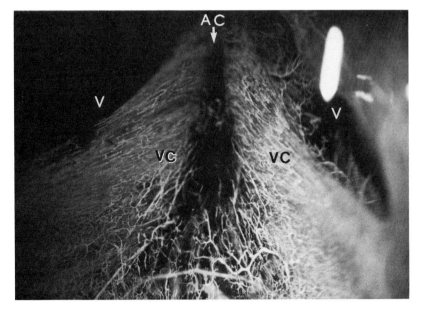

Fig. 6. Special injection technique demonstrates the glottic flow of blood vessels in an anterior/posterior direction. AC = Anterior commissure; V = ventricle; VC = vocal cord.

Table I. Spread of glottic tumour

---

(1) Arises from anterior portion of the membranous vocal cord
(2) Spreads horizontally along the cord in the mucosa
(3) Muscular invasion at site of origin and subglottic spread
(4) Spreads across the ventricle to involve the supraglottis
(5) At the same time tends to involve the anterior commissure
(6) Musculature of cord involved
(7) Spreads posteriorly and may be medial or lateral to the vocal process of the arytenoid
(8) Spreads beyond the larynx
    (1) Thyroid cartilage invasion at the anterior commissure
    (2) Spread through the anterior crico thyroid membrane
    (3) Spread through the lateral crico thyroid membrane
    (4) Posterial and lateral supraglottic escape
    (5) Vascular and perineural escape

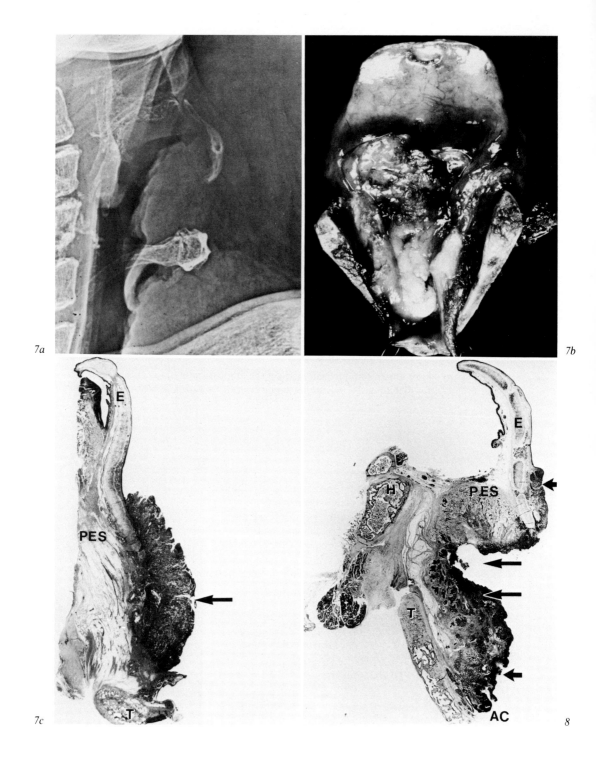

7a

7b

7c

8

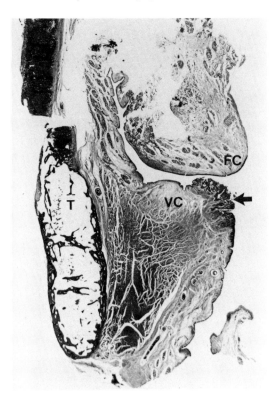

Fig. 9. This coronal section of the larynx in its anterior third, demonstrates a small isolated, glottic tumour which has remained very localized (black arrow). FC = False cord; VC = vocal cord; T = thyroid ala.

Fig. 7. a This lateral radiograph of the neck demonstrates the posterior surface of the infrahyoid epiglottis to be involved with tumour which does not extend to the anterior commissure and does not extend to the free tip of the epiglottis. *b* This operative picture is viewed from the posterior aspect to illustrate the large supraglottic tumour involving the posterior surface of the epiglottis as described in *a* and *c*. This sagittal section of the same tumour illustrates the localization of the malignancy to the posterior surface of the epiglottis. This is the most common site for supraglottic tumour. E = Epiglottis; PES = pre-epiglottic space; T = thyroid ala. The black arrow is pointing to the tumour.

Fig. 8. This sagittal section of the larynx at the level of the epiglottis (E), demonstrated by the black arrows, is a supraglottic tumour involving the epiglottis, invading the pre-epiglottic space (PES) and appearing in the floor of the vallecula. H = Hyoid bone; T = thyroid cartilage; AC = anterior commissure.

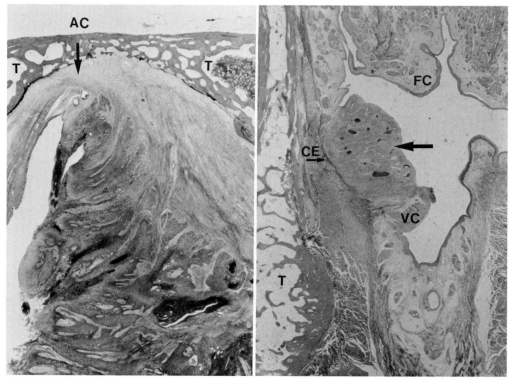

10   *11*

Fig. 10. A horizontal section of the tumour approaching the anterior commissure (AC) showing the anterior commissural tendon which prevents tumour spread to the opposite side. T = Thyroid cartilage.

Fig. 11. This coronal section at the anterior commissure demonstrates the obstruction to spread inferiorly at the anterior commissure by the conus elasticus (CE). FC = False cord; VC = vocal cord; T = thyroid alae; arrow = anterior commissure carcinoma.

carried out. Invasion of the thyroid cartilage with its destruction and the extension of the tumour through the crico-thyroid muscle is a common escape route for the anteriorly placed tumours (fig. 15). The surgeon should therefore remove a wedge of skin which covers the area of the crico-thyroid membrane in these cases as the tumour may be subcutaneous.

Lateral escape through the crico-thyroid space is also common (fig. 16), and this area should not be skeletonized at surgery. Posteriorly, the inter-arytenoid muscle may be involved and the tumour be sub-

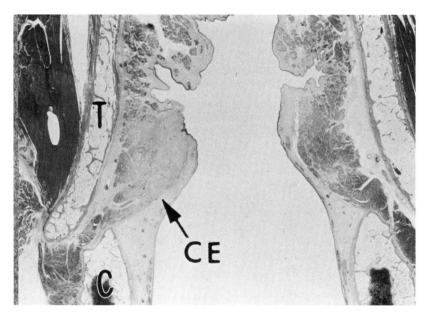

Fig. 12. Coronal section of a radiated case shows a glottic tumour which has been replaced by fibrous tissue and demonstrates the barrier action of the conus elasticus (CE). T = Thyroid alae; C = cricoid cartilage.

mucosal on the postcricoid area (fig. 14). When the crico-pharyngeal sphincter is being preserved at total laryngectomy, the danger of submucosal spread in this area must be appreciated in order to avoid leaving tumour behind which may subsequently result in stomal recurrence.

Supraglottic Tumour Spread (table II)

The site of predelection for supraglottic tumours is the laryngeal surface of the infra-hyoid epiglottis (fig. 7). Tumours tend to remain localized to this area for some time and do not readily extend inferiorly to invade the anterior commissure. This is the basis for the successful development of the conservation technique of supraglottic laryngectomy.

Tumours arising from the epiglottis tend to destroy the cartilage and invade the pre-epiglottic space (fig. 17). From this position, invasion of the paraglottic space is common where no barriers exist to the spread of tumour (fig. 18).

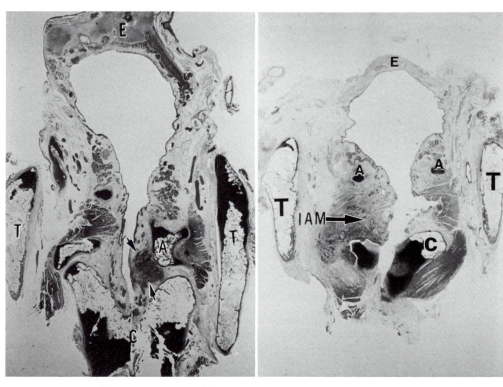

13 *14*

Fig. 13. A coronal section taken through a posterior aspect of the larynx to demonstrate tumour (arrows) under intact mucosa and lying medial to the arytenoid cartilage (A). T = Thyroid alae; E = epiglottis.

Fig. 14. A coronal section more posteriorly placed than figure 13 demonstrating tumour involving intra-arytenoid muscle (IAM) and destroying arytenoid (A) and cricoid cartilage (C) posteriorly. E = Epiglottis; T = thyroid alae.

Table II. Supraglottic spread

(1) Tumours of epiglottis invade the cartilage and extend into the pre-epiglottic space
(2) Bilateral extension to invade the false cords but rarely the glottis
(3) False cord tumours spread forwards to invade the epiglottis and the pre-epiglottic space
(4) Backwards to the arytenoid to become glottic and subglottic
(5) Upwards to the aryepiglottic fold
(6) Suprahyoid epiglottic tumours destroy cartilage and spread to base of tongue
(7) Aryepiglottic tumours spread downward to the false cord and laterally to pyriform sinus mucosa
(8) Outside the larynx anteriorly, laterally and posteriorly

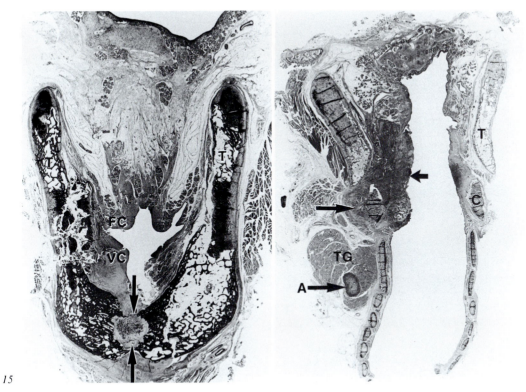

Fig. 15. A coronal section at the anterior commissure to demonstrate invasion of the thyroid ala (T) by an anteriorly placed glottic carcinoma (arrows) which is extending into the tissues of the anterior neck. FC = False cord; VC = vocal cord; T = thyroid cartilage.

Fig. 16. A coronal section of the larynx to demonstrate the escape of tumour (arrows) through the crico-thyroid space. A small adenoma of the thyroid gland is noted (arrow A). T = Thyroid cartilage; C = cricoid cartilage; TG = thyroid gland.

Carcinomas arising in the supra-hyoid epiglottis may be localized to the tip (fig. 19) and are highly curable. As these tumours enlarge, they destroy the epiglottis and invade the vallecula and extend to the base of the tongue (fig. 20). It is this anterolateral spread of tumours to the tongue which is difficult to detect clinically and which make conservation surgery hazardous.

False cord tumours are not common, but when they occur they may occasionally invade the glottis (fig. 21), and also will reach the paraglottic space and spread forward to the pre-epiglottic area. Spread to the glottis usually precludes the use of supraglottic laryngectomy in these cases.

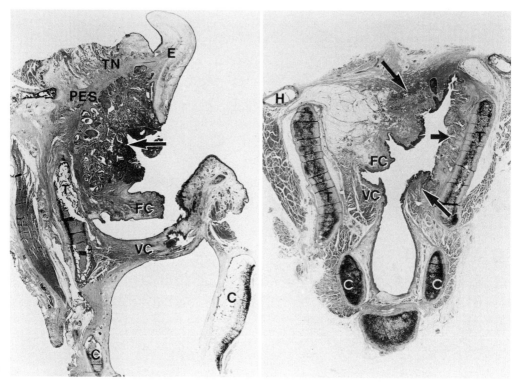

17

18

Fig. 17. A sagittal section of the larynx to illustrate the destruction of the posterior surface of the epiglottis (E) by a tumour which is extending into the pre-epiglottic space (PES). TN = Tongue; T = thyroid alae; FC = false cord; VC = vocal cord; C = cricoid cartilage.

Fig. 18. A coronal section well forward in the larynx to demonstrate the spread of tumour (arrows) in the pre-epiglottic space to the paraglottic space. H = Hyoid bone; FC = false cord; VC = vocal cord; C = cricoid cartilage.

Trans-glottic tumours have been variously described but this term should be restricted to describe a clinical entity where the malignancy is deeply invasive and spreads extensively in the paraglotic space, perhaps arising in the ventricle. The tumour spreads beneath intact mucosa and multiple biopsies are needed to make the diagnosis. Clinically, the patient presents with a frozen hemi-larynx without gross evidence of tumour. The tomogram is typical (fig. 22). In figure 23, the extensive trans-glottic spread is apparent. This type of laryngeal tumour has a poor prognosis and should be recognized as a clinical entity to allow

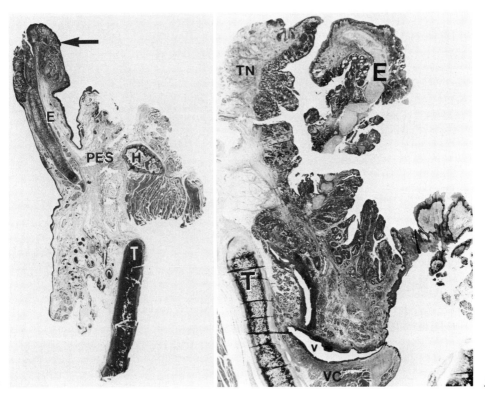

Fig. 19. A sagittal section of the larynx to demonstrate involvement of the tip of the epiglottis (E) by tomour (arrow). This tumour is isolated to the tip of the epiglottis. PES = Pre-epiglottic space; H = hyoid bone; T = thyroid cartilage.

Fig. 20. A sagittal section of the larynx demonstrating the involvement of the valleculae by supraglottic tumour which has destroyed the epiglottis (E). TN = Tongue; T = thyroid cartilage; V = ventriculus; VC = vocal cord.

for earlier diagnosis. In figure 23 an island of free tumour lying in the tissue outside the larynx is highly significant of the aggressiveness of this particular cancer.

Knowledge of the clinically significant anatomy of the larynx is best gained by the study of whole organ serial sections of the larynx. Study of surgical specimens by the same technique allows the surgeon to be familiar with the usual pathways of tumour spread and thus develop a third dimensional view of the extent of the tumour in any given case.

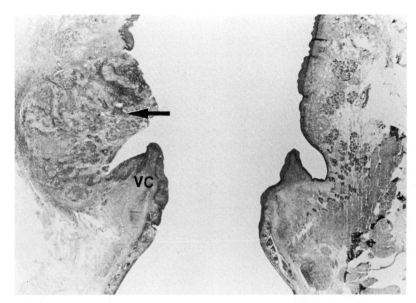

Fig. 21. A coronal section demonstrating a false cord tumour (arrow) which has extended inferiorly to involve the vocal cord (VC).

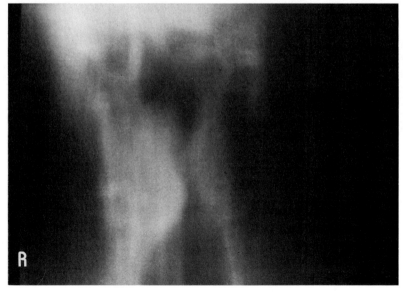

Fig. 22. A laryngeal tomogram demonstrating on the right side a uniform thickening of the larynx which involves the supraglottis, glottis and subglottis with distortion of the subglottic space. R = Right.

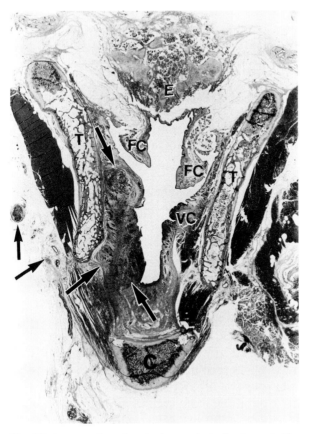

Fig. 23. A coronal section to demonstrate the transglottic nature of the tumour (long arrows) shown to involve the supraglottis, glottis and subglottis. The short arrows point to spread of tumour outside the larynx within lymphatic channels and a lymph node. E = Epiglottis; FC = false cord; T = thyroid cartilage. VC = vocal cord; C = cricoid cartilage.

Acknowledgments

Mrs. *Janice Etty* and Mr. *Ken Ekem* prepared the histologic sections. Miss *Alison MacKay* and the Medical Photography Department of the Toronto General Hospital prepared the illustrations.

Dr. D.P. Bryce, Department of Otolaryngology, University of Toronto, 92 College Street, Toronto M5S 1A1 (Canada)

Adv. Oto-Rhino-Laryng., vol. 29, pp. 24–26 (Karger, Basel 1983)

Problems in Classification of Some Head and Neck Tumours

D.F.N. Harrison

Institute of Laryngology and Otology, University of London, London, England

The purposes of classification are many but primarily serve to facilitate exchange of information between treatment centres and to assist in planning therapy. Even if it were possible for each and every clinician to objectively assess any specific tumour with complete accuracy, some sites are more accessible than others. Although there is a common value in the usage of all systems of classification, increased accuracy of record keeping, there are considerable inherent inaccuracies in the clinical application for most sites within the head and neck. Since new and existing treatment modalities, together with retrospective and prospective analysis, are usually based upon information gained by the application of such classification systems – the possibility of considerable but unknown errors are enormous. Awareness of such deficiencies is some compensation but only the introduction of site classifications that relate to known natural behaviour will produce reliable results.

An obvious omission from most systems is the histological type of the tumour. Within the larynx it is well established that anaplastic carcinomata at any site have a worse prognosis than well-differentiated tumours. Intrinsic growth rate and the tumour-host relationship cannot yet be estimated yet markedly influences prognosis. All systems are based on often ill-defined anatomical sites and regions although malignant tumours are no respecters of such boundaries. Since the underlying purpose of classification is to obtain homogeneous, statistically equivalent groups of patients, such errors may destroy the credibility of many supposed new innovations in therapy. All systems are clinically orientated and as such are dependent upon the clinical expertise and integrity of the reporting clinician. Can the clinician evaluate objectively the available information with sufficient accuracy? For many sites this may be difficult if not impossible.

With early laryngeal cancer, tumour definition is reasonably precise although the true limitations of the vocal cord were only agreed upon in 1974! As the tumour grows in size or infiltrates laryngeal structures the problems in describing a three-dimensional disease two dimensionally increases. A recent evaluation of 145 serially sectioned whole organ sections from total laryngectomies, staged clinically and then pathologically shows that on 5-year follow-up prognosis is primarily related to whether regional lymph node metastases are present or whether tumour has extended outside the laryngeal framework. It is possible that by utilizing a complex and often very inaccurate system of classification, we deceive ourselves as to the significance of much of the T stages. A further example of early glottic carcinoma amply illustrates the inbuilt confusion in the present UICC classification system for the larynx. The 5-year cure rate for T_1N_0 glottic is 72%. However, these cases include a proportion of T_1b tumours which at worse may extend from one vocal process across the anterior commissure to the controlateral vocal cord. Depending upon the proportion of these more serious T_1b lesions (a crude 5-year survival rate of 65%), individual T_1N_0 results may vary from 85 to 65%!

Within the maxillary sinus the problem is greater since tumour extent is largely determined radiologically. The more sophisticated the equipment the more accurate the T estimation. As yet the UICC have not agreed on a system but those utilized by the USA and Japan bear little relationship to the known natural history of sinus cancer. Regional and systemic metastases are uncommon and prognosis largely depends upon local control. Consequently, those tumours occurring in accessible regions such as facial skin are resectable – and potentially curable. Those extending to apex of orbit, nasopharynx or pyterygopalatine fossa are invariably not resectable and if not cured by radiotherapy – and they are usually not – lead to a poor prognosis.

In establishing a classification system for the maxillary sinus, increasing T numbers should be related to such known factors, i.e.:

T_1 Tumour confined to the maxillary sinus with no evidence of bony involvement.

T_2 Bony erosion without evidence of involvement of facial skin, orbit, pyterygopalatine fossa or ethmoidal labyrinth.

T_3 Involvement of orbit, ethmoidal labyrinth or facial skin.

T_4 Tumour extension to nasopharynx, sphenoidal sinus or pyterygopalatine fossa.

The development of craniofacial techniques will possibly allow early involvement of cribriform plate to be effectively resected allowing such lesions to remain as T_3. Similarly, criticisms can be applied to the floor of the mouth and hypopharynx and in evaluating treatment reports particularly advocating new treatment modalities, it is wise to bear in mind these intrinsic weaknesses which can easily be responsible for what may appear to be a major breakthrough in cancer management.

D.F.N. Harrison, MD, Institute of Laryngology and Otology, University of London, 330 Gray's Inn Road, London WC 1 (England)

Adv. Oto-Rhino-Laryng., vol. 29, pp. 27–38 (Karger, Basel 1983)

Current Management of Laryngotracheal Injury

Douglas P. Bryce

Department of Otolaryngology, University of Toronto, and Toronto General Hospital, Toronto, Ont., Canada

In the past 20 years, the problems of management of injury to the laryngotracheal complex have changed greatly, due chiefly to the improvements in management of patients admitted to intensive care units in our hospitals. Whereas previously, injuries to the trachea were commonly seen as a result of inflated endotracheal tube cuffs to allow for positive pressure respiration, these are now rare. Injuries from endotracheal tubes almost exclusively now involve the larynx and the immediate subglottis.

Direct trauma to the larynx and trachea as a result of gunshot and knife injuries as well as accidents involving automobiles, snowmobiles and dune buggies produces a constant number of very acute injuries which require expert, acute and chronic care for their proper management.

Lesions Due to Direct Trauma

The current spectrum of laryngotracheal injuries due to direct trauma include supraglottic fractures, lateral glottic fractures, or a combination of these, and cricotracheal separation.

Supraglottic and Lateral Glottic Fractures

The management of these injuries is greatly simplified if diagnosis can be made early. This is usually difficult as such injuries are almost always associated with damage to the brain, spine or chest which must take precedence in the treatment protocol. Only later, will the injury to the larynx or trachea be noted usually because of airway obstruction

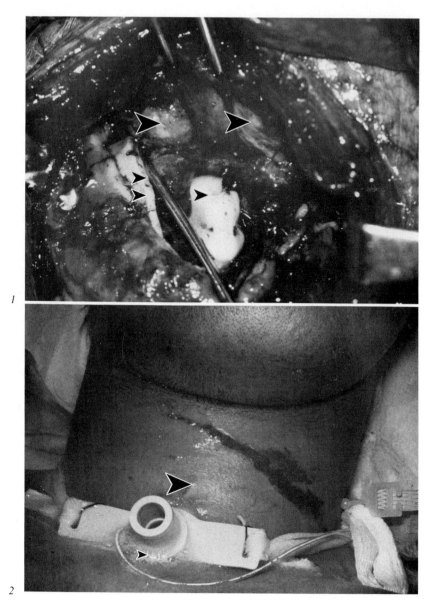

Fig. 1. This operative photograph illustrates the injury as seen when the larynx was first opened. A normal-looking glottis is occupied by an indwelling silastic stent (small black arrow). The free edge of the torn thyroid alae is seen on the right side (2 small black arrows). The remainder of the supraglottis consisting of the superior portions of the thyroid alae and the aryepiglottic folds are seen superiorly (large black arrows).

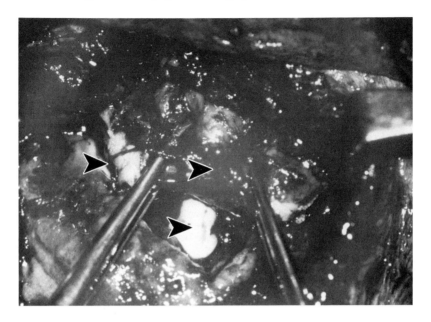

Fig. 3. The supraglottis is being pulled inferiorly into the appropriate position by two forceps. The indwelling silastic prothesis can be seen (inferior large black arrows) and the supraglottis (superior large black arrow) is being pulled forward and downward with some difficulty to be sutured to the inferior portion of the larynx which will restore the normal laryngeal structure.

and because extubation may not be possible. Early diagnosis can only be achieved if the presence of laryngotracheal injury is suspected due to the nature of the accident and the type of associated injuries.

Supraglottic fracture results in fracture and displacement of the supraglottic structure superiorly and posteriorly (fig. 1). In the male, diagnosis of this injury may be suspected when a flattening of the anterior cartilagenous structures of the neck is observed (fig. 2).

When managed acutely, the displaced structures can be relatively easily reduced through an anterior approach (fig. 3). This is best done about an individually moulded stent to provide support and stability to

Fig. 2. In this male patient who has a marked supraglottic fracture, the normal prominance of the tyroid alae is lost (large black arrow) and saliva is seen issuing from the tracheotomy indicating the presence of free aspiration because of laryngeal disruption (small black arrow).

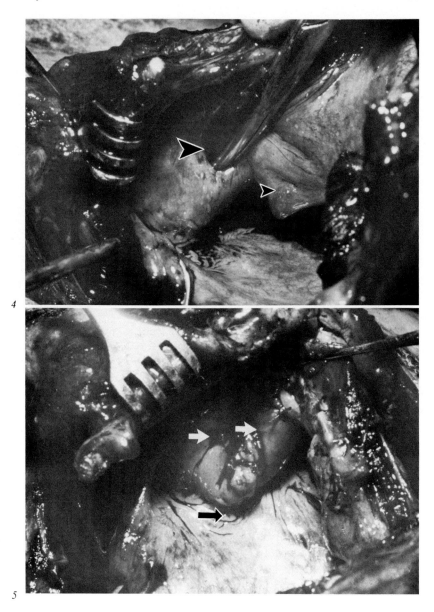

Fig. 4. The forcep is in the entrance to the supraglottis and a well-formed completely circumferential supraglottic stricture is outlined (large black arrow). The displaced epiglottis is illustrated (small black arrow).

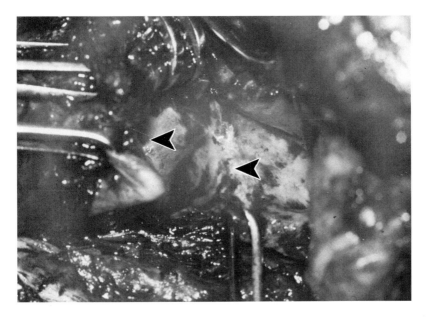

Fig. 6. This is a view of the larynx, posterior pharyngeal wall and hypopharynx as seen through a lateral pharyngotomy. The strictured laryngeal inlet lies in the direction of the 3 forceps (black arrow) and at the point of the single inferior forcep the pharyngeal scarring is seen (black arrow).

the larynx in the postoperative stage. Such early repair will result in the restoration of a normal larynx.

Supraglottic fracture if unrecognized in the acute phase will often be misdiagnosed when the varying degrees of supraglottic strictures result later. The displaced epiglottis often hides the stricture to mirror view and the direct laryngoscope may lift the scar tissues out of the way and make diagnosis difficult.

In figure 4, a well-developed supraglottic stricture is demonstrated through a lateral pharyngeal approach. Surgical excision of the scarred supraglottis with lateral mucous advancement for repair is the procedure of choice (fig. 5). The amount of the supraglottic structures which must be removed will vary with the extent of the stricture.

Fig. 5. The post-cricoid area of the hypopharynx is illustrated (black arrow). Repair of the denuded supraglottic area by advancement of hypopharyngeal mucosa from the piriform sinuses can be seen (white arrows).

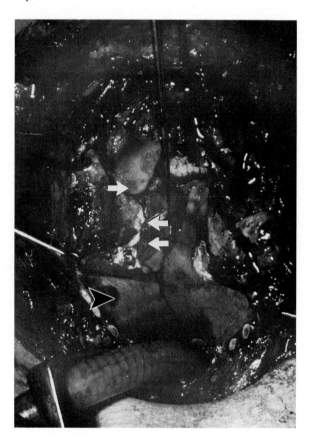

Fig. 7. This operative photograph illustrates a severe cricotracheal separation. The endotracheal tube can be seen entering the distal trachea (single large black arrow). Fractured fragments of the cricoid cartilage are illustrated (superior large white arrow). The torn posterior tracheal wall mucosa, which has been avulsed from the cricoid cartilage superiorly, lies inferiorly (2 white arrows).

Although direct trauma is the most common cause of supraglottic stricture, other injuries may produce the same clinical picture. In figure 6 a stricture of the supraglottis can be seen as well as a scarred posterior pharyngeal wall. This resulted from successful radiation for a malignant lesion of the lateral pharyngeal wall 12 years previously. Treatment in these cases is much more complicated as the blood supply to the larynx and pharynx is grossly comprised by the previous radiation. The principles of management, however, remain the same.

Although the supraglottic area is usually approached by supra-hyoid or lateral pharyngeal routes, stricture of the supraglottis may also be managed by an anterior thyrotomy approach.

Lateral glottic fracture is a well-recognized clinical entity in which there is fracture of the thyroid alae in the vertical plane and the ipsilateral vocal and arytenoid are torn and denuded. Such an injury is best managed by an anterior laryngo-fissure approach with excision of the damaged or scarred components of the glottis and mucosal repair as indicated.

Occasionally, there will be a combination of the lateral and supraglottic fractures. In these cases, the disruption of the mucosa of the cord, usually with displacement of the arytenoid, may extend to the ary-epiglottic folds and the epiglottis and result in complete airway obstruction because of a later-developing supraglottic stricture. Such strictures are best managed by the anterior thyrotomy approach by which the scarring of the cord can be excised and repaired and the supraglottic stricture also excised. The epiglottis may be freed and displaced anteriorly into its normal position and skin or mucous membrane of the hypopharynx may be used to repair the denuded areas.

Such an injury should be supported by the insertion of a moulded silastic laryngeal stent to allow mucosal healing without further scar formation. Very commonly, interarytenoid scarring may complicate the healing process and further excision of this may be necessary by cautery or the use of laser. A further complication will be the immobility of the injured vocal cord and thus aspiration may be a problem in the postoperative period.

A variety of injuries may be associated in any serious trauma to the larynx. Bold and ample surgical exposure and repair is the key to successful management.

Laryngotracheal Separation

The only common traumatic injury to the trachea results in laryngotracheal separation at the level of the first tracheotomy ring. The cricoid ring is usually fractured anteriorly and the mucosa of the subglottis torn and displaced with the trachea into the superior mediastinum (fig. 7). Many of these patients die before tracheotomy can be carried out, although in some cases an airway may be maintained in the pre-

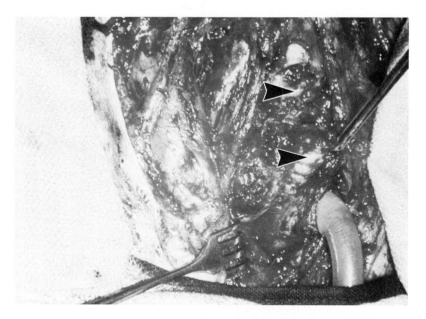

Fig. 8. A chronic laryngotracheal separation is illustrated. The posterior plate of the cricoid (superior arrow) and the scared distal retracted portion of the trachea (inferior arrow) are seen. There is a very great gap present here and considerable scarring.

sence of complete separation for 24 h. Usually, a tracheotomy is established into the open distal trachea as an emergency procedure and thus the diagnosis is made.

Repair must await control of infection and as a result, primary surgery may be delayed for up to 2 weeks. At surgery, the distal trachea is sutured to the cricoid plate and the stent is inserted to support the anastomosis and left in place for about 4 weeks. A distally placed tracheotomy is necessary. The recurrent laryngeal nerves will always be irreparably damaged in severe cases and no effort to repair them is justified.

Following successful primary repair of laryngotracheal separations, bilateral cord paralysis rarely results in airway obstruction. The position which the cords ultimately take up will change over a period of a year or more and usually the airway is adequate. False cord phonation replaces cordal approximation and a useful, husky voice will result.

In those cases in which primary repair has not been achieved, total subglottic stenosis inevitably results and must be managed by resection

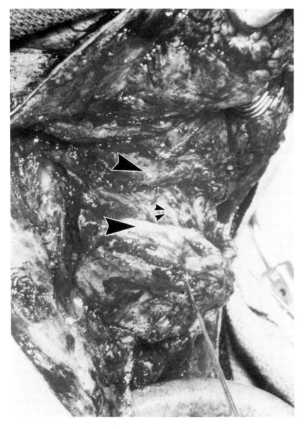

Fig. 9. This operative photograph illustrates a laryngeal drop carried out by an incision of the thyrohyoid membrane (2 small black arrows). The superior border of the thyroid alae (inferior large black arrow) and the hyoid bone (superior large black arrow) are illustrated. The endotracheal tube can be seen in the inferior aspect entering the trachea.

of the scar and direct anastomosis. Often the gap between the cricoid plate above and the trachea distally may be great (fig. 8). A laryngeal drop (fig. 9) is usually necessary and this combined with flexion of the head and careful freeing of the distal trachea will usually be successful in allowing approximation. An indwelling stent sutured above and below the line of anastomosis is mandatory in order to mould the disparate shape of the larynx above and the fracture below and also to support and strengthen the suture line of the anastomosis.

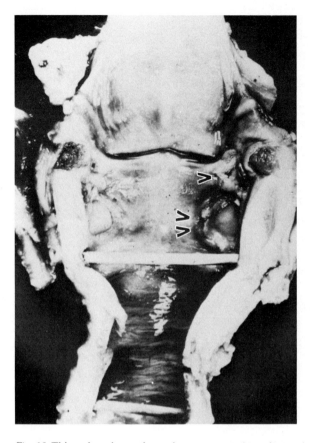

Fig. 10. This cadaveric specimen demonstrates ulceration at the vocal process of the arytenoid (single black arrow). Such ulceration frequently extends into the subglottis (2 black arrows). These injuries result from indwelling nasal or orotracheal tubes and result in subsequent posterior laryngeal scarring extending into the glottis.

Subglottic strictures resulting from laryngotracheal separation and cricoid fracture usually involve the immediate subglottic area. Excision of scars extending almost to the vocal cord subglottically is possible if the posterior plate of the cricoid cartilage is preserved and thinned to allow the distal trachea to be advanced anteriorly over the plate and the tracheal mucosa then sutured to the immediate subglottic mucosa. Inevitably, there will be damage to the laryngeal musculature in these cases and cord movement will be permanently impaired at some point in the postoperative period.

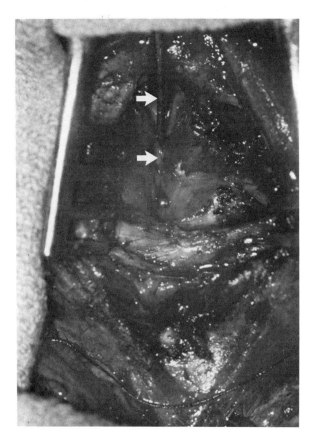

Fig. 11. This operative thyrotomy view of the larynx demonstrates an interarytenoid band under which the probe (white arrows) has been passed. Simple excision of this band is the solution to this problem.

Lesions Due to Intubation

Injuries to the laryngotracheal complex due to intubation are much less common, since the introduction (for positive pressure respiration assistance) of the large low-pressure cuffs on oral or nasopharyngeal tubes. The incidence of significant injury has dropped from 18% to 3% for those patients receiving positive pressure respiration and who have been successfully extubated. Moreover, the injuries that do occur affect the larynx primarily. A cadaveric specimen (fig. 10) demonstrates the sites of injury on the vocal process of the arytenoids and the posterior commissure. The scar will extend downward to involve the immediate subglottic area usually more severely to one side.

The simplest problem seen as a result of this injury is an interarytenoid band (fig. 11). This is readily managed by incision or by cautery or the use of laser. It is much more serious and difficult to manage if the posterior scar involves the posterior commissure itself and thus, over a period of weeks subsequent to extubation, gradually reduces the motion of the vocal cords until they become fixed in the midline and obstruct the airway. Diagnosis may be difficult and be confused with bilateral paralysis, unless the motility of the arytenoids is tested by direct laryngoscopy.

The surgical approach to correct this stenosis is by thyrotomy with excision of the scars in the posterior larynx and re-epithelialization either by skin or by mucosa of the denuded area. This procedure is usually successful, although the full mobility of the cords is almost never restored.

The frequency of laryngotracheal injury, as seen by the surgeon, has decreased in the past 10 years and the type of the injury has also changed. The problems seen today, however, are more difficult to treat and demand application of all the surgeon's skills for successful management.

Dr. D.P. Bryce, Department of Otolaryngology, University of Toronto, 92 College Street, Toronto M5S 1A1 (Canada)

Adv. Oto-Rhino-Laryng., vol. 29, pp. 39–49 (Karger, Basel 1983)

The Vertiginous Syndrome

W.J. Oosterveld

University of Amsterdam, Amsterdam, The Netherlands

Introduction

Vertigo is a symptom and not a disease. It is a disturbance in the orientation detecting system of a patient. Orientation can be defined as the ability of an individual to determine his position in the framework of his environment concerning accelerations, forces and visual fields. Orientation is derived from three main sources: the vestibular organs, vision and the propriocepsis in muscles and joints. The collected information is processed in the sensory integratory area in the reticular formation. The information processing under normal conditions and circumstances happens unconsciously. However, when the information contents parts that are new to the individual or that have an uncommon character, a condition is created under which the phenomenon vertigo can be generated.

The origin of vertigo is not restricted to the vestibular system only, it must be considered as part of an integration process that becomes conscious. Vertigo is the sensation of a movement pattern which is not in accordance with reality, it is an illusion.

The vertiginous patient senses movements, independent of the proper action of his balance organs. These sensations can be rotatory sensations, swing sensations, the sensation to be in an elevator or forward/backward movements. Vertigo is a symptom which accounts for about 5% of all consultations with a general practitioner. For patients examined by the otorhinolaryngologist, the incidence rate is reported to be 10–15% [*Rubin,* 1969]. The major cause for this high presentation rate is twofold. Firstly vertigo is a symptom which accompanies a large

number of complaints. A review by *Holt and Thomas* [1976] listed no
less than 69 causes of vertigo and even that was not exhaustive. Secondly, the term 'vertigo' is often used to describe a wide variety of subjective sensations. *Daroff* [1977] has given a strict definition of vertigo as
'an illusory sense of unidirectional environment and/or bodily rota-
tional movement'. In the English literature a difference is made between dizziness and vertigo. *Dorlands Medical Dictionary* defines dizziness as 'a disturbed sense of relationship to space; a sensation of unsteadiness with a feeling of movement within the head', and vertigo as
'a sensation as if the external world were revolving around the patient
or as if he himself were revolving in space'. However, the term tends to
be used, by patients and practitioner alike, to include a much wider
spectrum of sensations, from dizziness or disequilibrium through spa-
tial disorientation to simple faintness or light headedness. Specialists
in the field have repeatedly stressed the need for precision in describing
the patient's symptomatology if diagnosis, let alone treatment, is to be
successful [*Drachman and Hart,* 1972]. Nevertheless, because of frequent ambiguity in the patient's account of what he is experiencing and
also because of the real possibility that several 'vertiginous symptoms'
may be experienced together, it seems reasonable to regard many patients as suffering from a syndrome of symptoms which can perhaps
best be designated as the vertiginous syndrome. It must be noted that
making this designation does not necessarily make any assumptions
about possible relationships between the various causes which may un-
derly the patient's symptomatology. The term syndrome, in this connection, does not necessarily have any close bearing on the pathogene-
sis of the patients condition. Even less it is meant to represent a precise
diagnostic category. But it does seem a fair description of the complex
of true vertigo and associated symptoms of which many patients com-
plain.

The term vertiginous syndrome is not, however, completely without diagnostic value. Many different diagnostic schemes have been
used by different authors to encompass the causes of vertigo and related complaints. *Holt and Thomas* [1976], for example, organized their
69 causes of vertigo into seven categories from otologic to other. It is
clear from what has been said so far that no similar precise subdivision
would be claimed for diagnosing the causes of the vertiginous complex.
Nonetheless, it is helpful to divide the underlying pathology into four
categories.

The underlying complaint may firstly be peripheral, affecting the labyrinthine balance mechanism of the inner ear and such a complaint may be organic (e.g. tinnitus) or functional (e.g. motion sickness). Secondly, the defect may be in the proprioceptive system, which carries information about the body's position and orientation to the brain. The complaint can be caused by the visual system, and finally the complaint may be central, affecting the brain itself and either directly or indirectly influencing the vestibular nuclei or other centers responsible for the reception and integration of information about the body's position. Central complaints may either be functional or organic, although relatively little is known about the influence of truly functional brain effects on the body's equilibrium.

Dizziness is often accompanied by the following symptoms: irritation, headache, listlessness, sleep disturbances, memory disturbances, concentration disturbances, balance disturbances, lack of interest, and ear buzzing.

Besides an anamnesis specifically directed to vertigo, of course information is needed with regard to signs and symptoms in the field of ophthalmology, neurology and otology.

Since much of the research, both experimental and clinical, stretches back over nearly two decades, I make no attempt to give a comprehensive review of the syndrome or its response to drug treatment.

Classification of Vertigo

Vertigo has different types in which it can appear: paroxysmal vertigo, chronic vertigo, sudden-onset and slowly decreasing vertigo, and positional vertigo. In paroxysmal vertigo the complaints appear episodic, divided by free intervals. Chronic vertigo is usually less severe, but continuing over a long period sometimes with changes in intensity. The vertigo with a sudden onset, the acute vertigo, starts abruptly and thereafter decreases slowly in intensity. Positional vertigo means that either in a certain position, or in a movement toward a position the complaint appears. The vertigo anamnesis consists of six leading questions: (1) type of vertigo; (2) onset and development in the course of time; (3) provoking circumstances; (4) vegetative symptoms; (5) ear anamnesis, and (6) state of consciousness.

Table I. Peripheral vestibular vertigo

Diagnosis	Duration	Characteristics	Cause
Ménière's disease	minutes–days	irregular attacks of vertigo, with tinnitus, fluctuating hearing loss and vegetative symptoms	endolymphatic hydrops
Labyrinthine vascular accident	weeks	acute vertigo, with or without hearing impairment	labyrinthine ischemia
Acute labyrinthitis	days–weeks	acute vertigo, vegetative symptoms, hearing impairment and tinnitus	otitis media
Serous labyrinthitis	chronic	rotatory vertigo	chronic otitis media, sometimes fistule horizontal canal
Vestibular neuronitis	days–weeks	acute rotatory vertigo, vegetative symptoms	viral infection vestibular nerve
Eighth nerve neuritis	days–weeks	acute rotatory vertigo, vegetative symptoms, hearing impairment	viral infection eighth nerve
Labyrinthine concussion	days–months	positional or positioning vertigo, chronic vertigo	small inner ear lesions
Herpes zoster oticus	weeks	rotatory vertigo, vegetative symptoms, earache, vesicular eruption external ear canal and auricle, sometimes facial nerve paresis	Herpes infection inner ear
Paroxysmal positional vertigo	less than ½ min	positional vertigo	dysfunction semicircular canals
Vertigo of childhood	minutes	paroxysmal vertigo in children up to age 12, no vegetative symptoms, no hearing impairment	unknown
Motion sickness	days–weeks	rotatory vertigo and vegetative symptoms	uncommon acceleration pattern
Epidemic vertigo	weeks	acute rotatory vertigo, slowly diminishing	viral infection labyrinth
Intoxications: more than 200 agents		chronic vertigo	inner ear lesions

Table II. Central vestibular vertigo

Diagnosis	Duration	Characteristics	Cause
Vestibular encephalitis	days	acute rotatory vertigo, vegetative symptoms, eye muscle dysfunction, pyramid track dysfunction	cerebral viral infection
Multiple sclerosis	days–months	positional vertigo, balance dysfunction	sclerotic patches in brain and spinal cord
Tumour fossa posterior	minutes	positional vertigo	pressure on brainstem and cerebellum
Cerebellar vascular accident	weeks	acute, very severe vertigo, cerebellar dysfunction symptoms	lesion cerebellar artery
Acute vermis syndrome	minutes–hours	acute, severe vertigo	posterior inferior cerebellar artery occlusion
Wallenberg's syndrome	days–weeks	acute rotatory vertigo with vegetative symptoms, homolateral palate paralysis, trigeminal nerve paralysis, heterolateral sensibility dysfunction	posterior inferior cerebellar artery occlusion
Vertebrobasilar artery insufficiency	minutes–hours	paroxysmal vertigo, vegetative symptoms, neurological symptoms	vertebrobasilar artery insufficiency
Superior cerebellar artery syndrome	days–weeks	acute vertigo, vegetative symptoms, cerebellar hemiataxia, hypotonia, intention tremor, speech disturbances	superior cerebellar artery occlusion
Cerebral sclerosis	long lasting	giddiness, unsteadiness, sway movements	diminished cerebral blood supply
Pontocerebellar arachnoiditis (Bárány syndrome)	hours	attacks of rotatory vertigo, occipital headache, vegetative symptoms, dysfunction fourth, sixth, seventh and eighth nerve, cerebellar dysfunction	posterior fossa arachnoiditis
Migraine equivalent	hours	vertigo and one-sided headache, vegetative symptoms	migraine
Postcommotional vertigo	weeks–months	irregular giddiness, orthostatic influences, increasing by physical or psychical strain	vascular lesions in brainstem and cerebellum

Table III. Epileptic vertigo

Diagnosis	Duration	Characteristics	Cause
Temporal lobe epilepsy	seconds	acute attack of vertigo, gastric aura, followed by diminished consciousness or unconsciousness	focus temporal lobe
Vestibular epilepsy	seconds	absences, dizziness spells, no vestibular symptoms, EEG disturbances, nonprovokable	focus superior temporal gyrus
Vestibulogenic epilepsy	minutes	unconsciousness, dizziness spells, vestibular symptoms, no EEG disturbances, provokable	decreased epileptic stimulation threshold

Table IV. Nonvestibular vertigo

Diagnosis	Duration	Characteristics	Cause
Cervical vertigo	minutes	rotatory vertigo provoked by head movements, often headache and neckache	Irritation cervical posterior nerve roots, intermittent suppression vertebral artery
Orthostatic vertigo	seconds–minutes	blurring of vision, giddiness and sway movements	fast changes in blood pressure by changes in body position
Vertigo e stomacho laesa	hours	paroxysmal vertigo	intrathoracic and intra-abdominal organ diseases
Hyperventilation syndrome	minutes	rotatory vertigo, fear, sometimes provoked by stress situations	hyperventilation

The main question is: what causes vertigo. According to the origin, vertigo has four main sources: vestibular vertigo, central or peripheral; nonvestibular vertigo, and epileptic vertigo.

As so many diseases are able to provoke vertigo, it is unfeasible to mention them all. The most important diseases which can be accompanied by vertigo are set forth in the next tables: peripheral vestibular vertigo (table I); central vestibular vertigo (table II); epileptic vertigo (table III), and nonvestibular vertigo (table IV).

When the practitioner encounters vertigo as the main complaint in a patient, his approach is twofold. First he determines the type of vertigo, secondly he makes up to other complaints, especially with regard to vegetative symptoms and hearing impairment. This last approach is much more practical. The following entities can be distinguished:

Paroxysmal vertigo, without cochlear symptoms
1 Hyperventilation syndrome
2 Cervical vertigo
3 Vertebrobasilar artery insufficiency
4 Multiple sclerosis
5 Brain tumors

Paroxysmal vertigo, with cochlear symptoms
1 Ménière' syndrome
2 Ménière's disease
3 Lermoyez's syndrome
4 (Peri-)labyrinthitis
5 Cerebellopontine angle tumors
6 Cerebellopontine arachnoiditis (Bárány's syndrome)
7 Cogan's syndrome

Vertigo, which begins suddenly and decreases slowly, without hearing impairment
1 Vestibualr neuronitis
2 Cerebrovascular accident
3 Epidemic vertigo
4 Multiple sclerosis
5 Brain concussion

Vertigo, which begins suddenly and decreases slowly, with hearing impairment
1 Octavus neuritis
2 Labyrinthitis
3 Labyrinth concussion
4 Ramsay-Hunt syndrome

Chronic vertigo, without hearing impairment
1 Cerebral atherosclerosis
2 Cervical arthrosis
3 Hypoglycemia
4 Psychogenic vertigo
5 Multiple sclerosis

Chronic vertigo, with hearing impairment
1 Chronic otitis media
2 Cerebral atherosclerosis
3 Intoxications
4 Cerebellopontine angle tumors
5 Multiple sclerosis

Positional vertigo
1 Benign paroxysmal positional vertigo
2 Positioning vertigo
3 Orthostatic vertigo
4 Cerebellar lesions

Ocular vertigo
1 Ocular muscle paresis
2 Vision abnormalities
3 Optokinetic vertigo
4 Fear of height

In the context of this paper I am not able to discuss extensively many diseases accompanied by the symptom vertigo. However, I want to make a few exceptions.

With regard to paroxysmal vertigo the diagnosis Ménière's disease is often misused. The diagnosis should depend upon a triad of symptoms: fluctuating hearing loss with tinnitus and recruitment, paroxysmal vertigo and vegetative signs as nausea and vomiting, sweating and the sensation to be in a miserable condition. The ear pathology in this disease is not clear at all. Endolymphatic hydrops is not always found and furthermore in many cases endolymphatic hydrops was reported to be found in patients without any complaint about vertigo or hearing impairment. *Schuknecht* [1978] emphasized the fact that the histopathology of this disease had many questions yet unanswered.

In the European population 1 out of 2,500 suffers from Ménière's disease. The disease affects man and woman equally. The disease can appear in all age groups, however, most cases are seen between 40 and 60 years. In about 80% of the cases the disease affects both ears. A proper treatment is not yet available. In case of vertigo with very brief attacks, only a few seconds, the following causes must be considered: (1) migraine, (2) epileptic vertigo, (3) orthostatic vertigo, and (4) vertigo of childhood.

Benign paroxysmal vertigo is not a rare disease. The cause of the disease is not known. Head movements, most of the time in a specific direction out of a specific position, cause a rather severe vertigo which lasts only 5–30 s. Usually the disease disappears after a period of several months up to 1 year. Before the introduction of antibiotics, labyrinthitis was a very serious condition with a high rate of mortality. Nowadays a clear labyrinthitis is a rare condition. A less dramatic but probably more common picture is the occurrence of a serous labyrinthitis secondary to a chronic otitis media. Physical damage to the labyrinth is a cause of severe debilitating vertigo and sickness producing a picture of 'helpless misery' with only a few parallels in medicine. The misery is caused by the bombardment of the brain with signals from only one labyrinth which are not compensated for by similar messages from the other side, if one labyrinth is damaged or destroyed. For a long time, treatment depended simply upon waiting for the brain to succeed in compensating for this imbalance.

Treatment of Vertigo

Therapy of vertigo is primarily directed to eliminate the underlying cause. This sounds rational, however, in many cases the origin of the complaint in vertiginous patients does not become clear. Even with sophisticated examination methods the cause of the vertigo in about 50% of the cases will not show up. As stated in the Introduction, vertigo is a symptom and not a disease. The therapy of vertigo is per definition a symptomatic treatment. Although many different diseases have vertigo in their package of symptoms and signs, the therapy of vertigo does not differ extensively. A confusing factor is that in many patients vertigo continuously changes its character as well as its intensity. Basically three different ways are open in the approach of vertigo: (1) surgical methods, (2) adaptation methods, and (3) drug treatment.

Surgical methods mean section of the vestibular nerve and several methods used in the treatment of Ménière's disease. Adaptation methods are sometimes very useful. Cooksey [1945] made a schedule of head and body movements, especially for the treatment of traumatic-induced benign vertigo. Dix [1976] has described a series of head exercises to assist the adaptation process. Young patients need much less time for adaptation than older patients do. Posttraumatic vertigo and vertigo due to a sudden loss of vestibular function on one side benefit from this method. Paroxysmal vertigo cannot be treated this way. In many cases a drug treatment cannot be avoided. Prescriptions for drugs are given in 80% of all cases of vertigo. Concerning the effect of a drug, three modes of action must be considered: first there is a 'vestibular tranquillizer', second there is an action on the vestibuar nuclei and third there is a action as a cerebral vasodilatator. Basically one can state that chronic vertigo needs chronic treatment and episodic vertigo needs episodic treatment. In case of a sudden loss of the function of one peripheral labyrinth, drug treatment decreases the severity of the vertigo, however, the time needed for adaptation to the new condition will be lengthened. Vertigo, due to cerebrovascular insufficiency, needs drug therapy for a long time, sometimes many years. Of the peripheral vestibular causes for vertigo, Ménière's disease is well known. It makes sense to pay some attention to the treatment of this disease. Many surgical methods to treat Ménière's disease have been described in the last two decennia. Torok [1977] stated that a bewildering number of concepts and methods have been suggested as the best answers until the next claim of success shatters the popularity of earlier allegations.

As stated previously, the diagnosis Ménière's disease is often not justified. In my clinic I am very conservative in the treatment of this disease. Several drugs are to be used in the treatment of vertigo. Betahistine, cinnarizine (stugeron), dogmatil (sulpiride), nootropil (piracetam), and tanganil (d-l-leucine) are the drugs used most of the time. In many cases of Ménière's disease drugs give a rather good protection against attacks, and in case that attacks nevertheless come through, the severity is usually much lower. Sometimes a high dosage, which means triple of the normal one is needed for a period of several weeks. Cinnarizine in a dosage of 300 mg/day and betahistine in a dosage of 72 mg/day can be given for periods of many months. In order to cut off an attack, a good choice is a prescription of motilium (domperidone) suppositories of 60 mg each given 4 times daily. Two different medication modes can be applied: (1) drug treatment only when an attack appears and (2) drug treatment continuously. When less than two attacks occur in 1 month, the first mode can be used, however, when two or more attacks occur in 1 month the second mode has priority. The vertiginous syndrome is a challenge to the practitioner. Thanks to adaptation methods and modern drugs the doctor is able to provide patients with a better protection than in earlier days.

References

Cooksey, F.S.: Proc. R. Soc. *39:* 273 (1945).
Daroff, R.B.: Am. Family Physn *16:* 143 (1977).
Dix, M.R.: Practitioner *217:* 919 (1976).
Drachman, D.A.; Hart, C.W.: Neurology *22:* 232 (1972).
Holt, G.R.; Thomas, J.R.: Family Physn *14:* 84 (1976).
Rubin, W.: Mod. Treat. *6:* 594 (1969).
Schuknecht, H.F.: Ann. Otol. Rhinol. Lar. *87:* 61 (1978).
Torok, N.: Laryngoscope *87:* 1870 (1977).

Prof. Dr. W.J. Oosterveld,
Academisch Ziekenhuis bij de Universiteit
van Amsterdam, Academisch Medisch Centrum, ENT Department,
Meibergdreef 9, NL-1105 AZ, Amsterdam (The Netherlands)

Adv. Oto-Rhino-Laryng., vol. 29, pp. 50–59 (Karger, Basel 1983)

Early Diagnosis of Acoustic Tumors by Using Auditory-Evoked Brain Stem Response

Shozo Kawamura

Department of Otolaryngology, Juntendo University, School of Medicine, Tokyo, Japan

Introduction

Diagnosis of the acoustic tumor in the early stage is quite important, because the surgical approaches to acoustic tumor showed satisfactory improvement. Recently, among the diagnostic tools for the acoustic tumor in the early stage, auditory-evoked brain stem response (ABR) has been closed up not only by the otologists but also by the neurologists. This tendency is now prevailing all over the world. ABR is easily recordable because of the remarkable advance of medical electronics. However, if we want to apply ABR for the diagnosis of acoustic tumor correctly, the modalities of ABR both in the physiological and pathological situation have to be understood.

In this paper, the modalities of ABR have been demonstrated to contribute to the discussion of the early diagnosis of acoustic tumor.

Method

Figure 1 is the block diagram of ABR recording. ABR was recorded with the surface electrodes placed on the vertex and the ipsilateral mastoid with ground on the forehead. 1,000–2,000 sweeps were averaged at each stimulus setting. Each sweep was filtered between 100 and 2,500 Hz (24 dB/oct). The stimulus was the click with the intensity of 60–80 dB above the normal hearing threshold. The repetition rate was 10/s.

Results

ABR of 21 cases of acoustic tumor admitted to our hospital in the past 4 years could be classified into four types (fig. 2). Type I is the

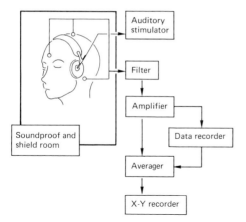

Fig. 1. The block diagram of ABR recording.

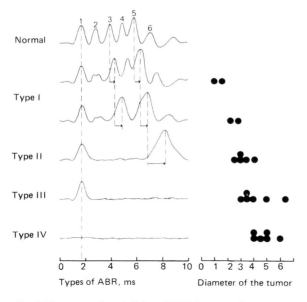

Fig. 2. The types of modalities of ABR in acoustic tumor.

prolongation I–III or I–V, and III–V interpeak latency, which is generally thought to be the modality of ABR in mid or upper brain stem lesion. Type II is only wave I and prolonged wave V. Type III is only wave I. Type IV is no response at all. On the right side of figure 2, the numbers in each type are shown with black dots, and the horizontal

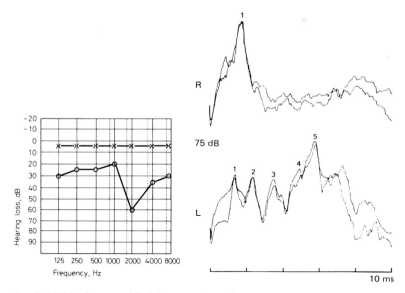

Fig. 3. ABR in the case with right acoustic neurinoma.

axis means the diameter of the tumors. Type I could be said to be the modalities of ABR of acoustic tumor in the early stage and type III or IV in the advanced stage.

The following 4 cases are the typical modalities of ABR in each pattern. Cases 1 and 2 are in the fairly advanced stage, and cases 3 and 4 are in the quite early stage of acoustic tumor.

Case 1: 53-Year-Old Woman. Her chief complaint was right hearing difficulty. Otoneurological findings revealed the right acoustic tumor. Figure 3 shows her audiogram and ABR. Only wave I could be detected in the affected side (type III), although the normal left side shows normal ABR. The tumor was surgically removed, which was 2.5 cm in diameter.

Case 2: 27-Year-Old Man. His chief complaint is left hearing difficulties. Otoneurologically, left acoustic tumor was suspected. Figure 4 shows his audiogram and ABR in which wave I and wave V with prolonged latency could be recognized on the left side (type II). The tumor was 2.0 cm in diameter. The modality of ABR with wave I and prolonged wave II could be obtained in fairly advanced acoustic tumors.

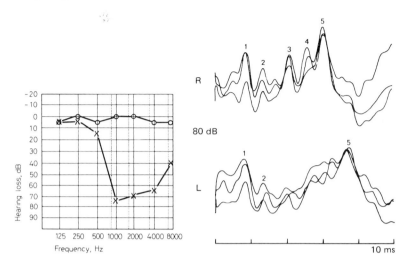

Fig. 4. ABR in the case with left acoustic tumor.

Case 3: 20-Year-Old Woman. The subject is one of the volunteers to do the control study of normal ABR variation with the newly purchased apparatus (signal processor). She was quite healthy and her hearing was normal. In the first trial, her ABR to right ear stimulation (fig. 5) showed prolonged I–III and I–V interpeak latency (type I).

At first we were surprised at such wide a normal variation. So she was retested five times on the same day, and each time the ABR showed the same pattern. Then on second thought, we came to the conclusion that the subject might have a certain dysfunction at the brain stem, even though there were no signs and no symptoms, except the radiological finding of the very slight enlargement of the inner ear canal at the affected side by 1 mm which should be said within normal variation.

We followed her ABR every month. Her 3-monthly ABR is shown in figure 6. ABR did not reveal any remarkable changes throughout the following year. 1 year 5 months after the initial ABR recording, she finally agreed to surgery, because the CT finding revealed fairly clear abnormalities at the c-p angle and at the same time she felt light tinnitus on the affected side. The tumor was surgically found about 1 cm in diameter.

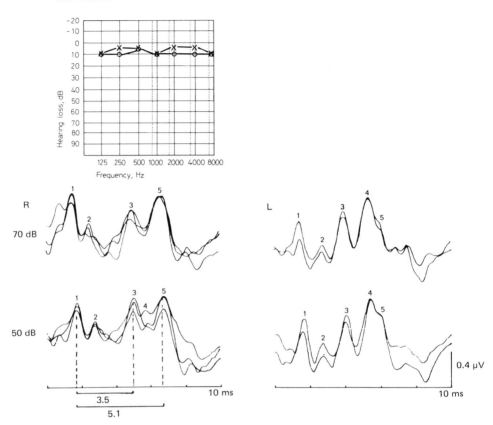

Fig. 5. ABR in the early stage of acoustic tumor.

Case 4: 47-Year-Old Woman. The chief complaints on her first visit to our clinic were tinnitus and hearing loss on the right side. Otoneurologically, no abnormal findings could be obtained and the initial examination of ABR (fig. 7) showed slight prolongation of III–V interpeak latency (type I), which suggested the upper brain stem lesion. No other abnormal findings could be obtained at this time.

On the second examination, not only wave I–V interpeak latency but also wave I–III interpeak latency showed remarkable prolongation as is shown in figure 7. At about this time, CT scanning showed the slight abnormal finding suspicious of acoustic tumor in quite an early stage. Surgical operation was performed and the tumor was 7 mm in di-

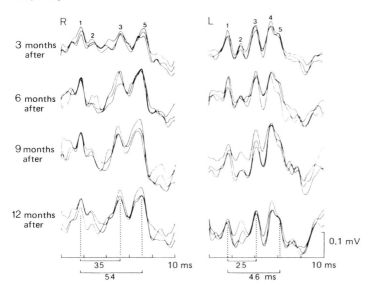

Fig. 6. ABR every 3 months in the case 3.

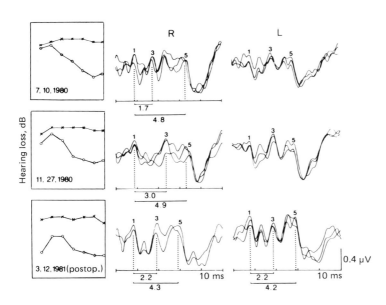

Fig. 7. ABR in the early stage of acoustic tumor.

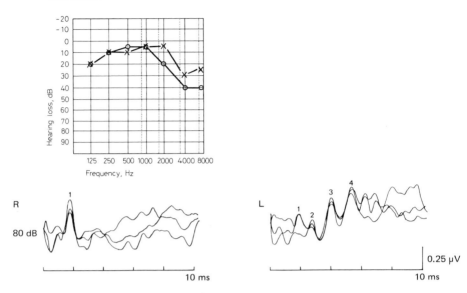

Fig. 8. ABR in the case of pontine glioma on the right side.

ameter. After surgery, the latency of waves III and V recovered into an almost normal range (fig. 7).

Discussion

Only a few reports on the ABR application for acoustic tumor have concluded that ABR was quite sensitive to the pathological situation of the 8th nerve [1–3]. However, general understanding of the abnormalities of waves III–V have much concern with the mid or upper brain stem [4]. In comparison with the above described acoustic tumors, 2 cases of brain stem tumor have been demonstrated here. Figure 8 shows a pontine glioma on the right side. On the contralateral side an almost normal pattern is seen.

Figure 9 is the case of another pontine glioma. In this case, the tumor located in the midportion and the ABR on both sides showed abnormal patterns. On the right side, waves IV and V disappeared, and on the left side, waves III–V disappeared. ABR is quite sensitive to the pathological condition of the 8th nerves and brain stem auditory pathway, but it is quite inadequate to mention the location of the lesion, on-

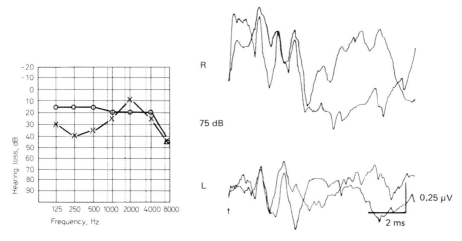

Fig. 9. ABR in the case of pontine glioma on the midline.

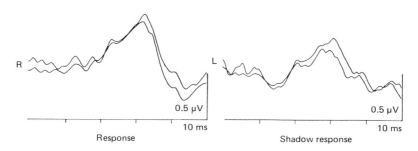

Fig. 10. Shadow response of the case with left unilateral deafness.

ly from the modality of ABR. Different kinds of tumor sometimes show a quite similar pattern of ABR. And when we discuss the modality of waves III–V, the shadow responses have to be ruled out carefully, because the morphology of shadow responses is quite similar to the true responses both in their latency and amplitude. The true responses are on the left side of figure 10 and shadow responses on the right in the unilateral deaf subject. 'R' and 'L' in each pair of traces mean that the responses were recorded the vertex-right and vertex-left mastoid tips respectively. The morphology of waves III–V reveals no remarkable variation between true and shadow responses. Generally, masking

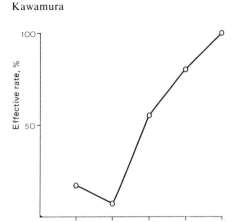

Fig. 11. Masking effect in ABR.

noise is applied to the nontested ear for the purpose of excluding the shadow responses.

The difficulty of masking the shadow responses was shown in figure 11. The horizontal axis means the intensity of the masking noise. Standard 0 dB is the intensity of the noise in order to mask the click of 30 dB psychoacoustically. The vertical axis means the effective rate of masking, and the solid line is ABR. This means that the shadow ABR could be excluded completely only when the masking noise more than 80 dB in n HL is applied to the nontested ear, and this is not necessarily impossible but quite a nuisance for the subjects. So, actually, we always have to think of the influence of the shadow responses upon the true ABR.

Conclusion

ABR is quite sensitive and reliable to detect the acoustic tumor in the early stage. The classification of the modalities of ABR in acoustic tumor in these studies leads us to the consider that we should not expect the specific patterns of ABR for acoustic tumor. None of the abnormal modalities of ABR could exclude acoustic tumor as one of the candidates for differential diagnosis.

References

1 Starr, A.; Achor, L.J.: Auditory brainstem response in neurological disease. Neurology *32:* 761–776 (1975).
2 House, J.W.; Brackman, D.E.: Brainstem audiometry in neurological diagnosis. Archs Otolar. *105:* 305–309 (1979).
3 Terkildsen, K.; Osterhammel, P.; Thomsen, J.: The ABR and MLR in patients with acoustic neuromas. Scand. Audiol. *13:* suppl., pp. 103–107 (1982).
4 Stokard, J.J.; Stockard, J.E.; Sharbrough, F.W.: Brainstem auditory evoked potentials in neurology; in Aminoff, Electrodiagnosis in clinical neurology, pp. 370–413 (Churchill Livingstone, Edinburgh 1980).

S. Kawamura, MD, Department of Otolaryngology, Juntendo University, School of Medicine, 2-1-1 Hongo, Bunkyo-Ku, Tokyo 113 (Japan)

Adv. Oto-Rhino-Laryng., vol. 29, pp. 60–67 (Karger, Basel 1983)

Diagnosis of Acoustic Neurinomas

K. Terkildsen, P. Osterhammel, J. Thomsen

ENT Department, Rigshospitalet, Copenhagen, Denmark

Looking back through the history of audiology it is impressive how much energy has been devoted to the recognition of retrocochlear disease and the diagnosis of cerebellopontine angle tumors. During the years a considerable number of procedures have been introduced and heralded as having a particularly high diagnostic specificity. In small series of patients they have identified nearly all tumors, but very few of these tests have stood the test of time and the general pattern has been that in large series about one third of the tumors would go undetected. During the same period operative techniques have improved, and it is now an absolute demand that the presence of such tumors should be recognized even when they are very small.

The experience from large series of patients clearly show that no single test will satisfy this demand, and it is necessary to use some combination of test procedures. It has been attempted [*Thomsen* et al., 1981] to evaluate this situation by means of complex statistical methods in order to decide which combination should be preferred. It is not surprising that certain tests rate very high in such an analysis: tomography of the internal auditory meatus, caloric vestibular examinations, the classical alternate binaural loudness balance (ABLB) test and its equivalent, the objective Metz recruitment test, and then the auditory brainstem responses (ABR), which I shall discuss in more detail later. One problem with such an analysis is that test results have to be rated as being either tumor-positive or tumor-negative. There is no room for uncertainties.

As a clinician I have been involved in the diagnosis of almost 150 neurinomas during the last 5 years, where for parsimonious reasons we gradually have eliminated all but a very few tests and now rely only on the above-named procedures. It has been interesting to notice how such a rather rigid approach tends to defeat itself. In the above-mentioned statistical analysis, tomography of the meatus came out as the most valid procedure. Denmark is a small country; the word goes around, and we now receive a number of patients for further diagnostic procedures, where radiologists from other institutions, who do not have the same experience, will describe tomograms – often of inferior quality – as being abnormal. We can also see how such a positive finding may cause a remarkable bias in the evaluation of subsequent tests. Such biasing effects are noticeable also with the ABLB and the classical Hallpike caloric procedure as clear evidence of the fact that most of our examinations contain considerable subjective elements.

A partial solution to this problem might be to have the examiner give a verbal statement about the confidence with which he has been able to interpret the results, but naturally it would be best only to use objective measurements. This is a main reason why we gradually have come to rely so much on the ABR in these patients [*Terkildsen* et al., 1981]. It is an excellent screening test and so far we have had only one truly false-negative finding. This was in a patient who had almost normal hearing and where, during surgery, the acoustic nerve was only attached to the capsule without being involved in the tumor process itself. It is not possible to give a meaningful figure for the number of false-positive findings, because it tests the function of the afferent auditory pathways and not the specific condition, where there is a mass in the cerebellopontine angle, so among the so-called false-positive findings there are patients with multiple sclerosis and brainstem lesions of various kinds.

In our routine we now combine the ABR with tomograms and caloric testing. If two or three of these tests are positive for tumor, we will obtain a CT scan and if this is negative for tumor the patients are submitted to computer tomography pneumocisternography (CT with air). If only one test is positive the patient will be seen again after 1 year, and if all three are negative, we diagnose the patient as not having a tumor. It should also be noticed that if the patient exhibits the presence both of loudness recruitment, normal caloric responses, and normal ABR, this will suffice to exclude the possibility of a tumor, and it is unnecessary to obtain tomographs.

With all these examinations a main problem has been to improve the technical quality. For the ABR much has already been attained in

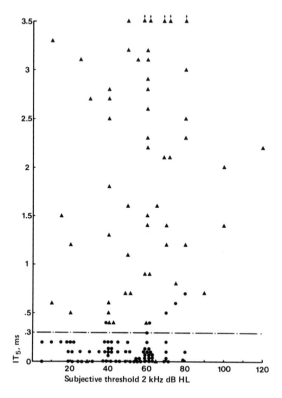

Fig. 1. IT$_5$ values in 56 neurinoma cases (▲) and 71 patients with Ménière's disease (●). Along the abscissa are individual, audiometric thresholds on the pathological ear at 2 kHz. 2 neurinoma patients are shown as having a normal IT$_5$; 1 of these was found very early in our series and it was later shown to represent an erroneous interpretation of the recording.

this respect. One problem is that so many of these patients have severely impaired hearing and particularly in the high frequencies. In the literature there is a good deal of disagreement on how this may influence the wave V latency. Quite undoubtedly the frequency characteristics of the sound transducer is important in this respect. For many reasons it has as yet not been possible to establish standard requirements to acoustic transducers that are used during ABR testing and the commercially available systems are certainly quite different in this respect.

    To some extent the acoustic spectrum that is delivered at the eardrum can be controlled by means of using sine waves to activate the

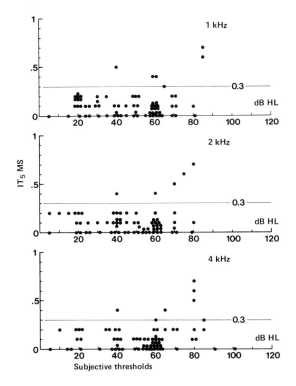

Fig. 2. The influence of hearing thresholds on the IT_5 in 71 patients with unilateral Ménière's disease. Along the abscissa are audiometric thresholds on the pathological ear for the frequencies that are indicated to the upper right for each graph.

transducer. This will increase the power density spectrum at the particular sine wave frequency with about 10 dB. Our general routine has been to use a full 2-kHz sine wave beginning in the rarefaction mode, but if the patient has a pronounced high frequency hearing loss, we may go to 1 kHz or even 0.5 kHz. Our measuring criterion is the wave V latency difference between the two sides, the so-called IT_5, and if we use the same stimulus at both ears this difference should remain the same.

Figure 1 shows IT_5 values for 56 neurinoma patients and 71 patients with Ménière's disease. Along the abscissa are the individual subjective audiometric thresholds at 2 kHz on the pathological ear, and the ordinate gives the magnitude of IT_5 in milliseconds. If the hearing at 2 kHz is poorer than 60 dB HL some patients in the Ménière group will

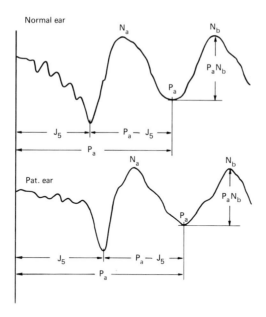

Fig. 3. Schematic illustration of the MLR and the parameters that were submitted to a statistical analysis.

produce an IT_5 that exceeds our 0.3 ms criterion for normality, but in other individuals such severe losses are still compatible with completely normal IT_5 values.

Figure 2 illustrates the importance of other audiometric frequencies in the same group of 71 Ménière patients. In the upper part the figures along the abscissa give the subjective audiometric thresholds at 1 kHz and below that are the results that were obtained when the thresholds on the pathological ear were measured at 2 and 4 kHz. It is apparent that with our technique the individual audiometric configuration does not cause any systematic changes in the IT_5.

Another troublesome problem may be the precise identification of wave V. During the last couple of years we have included the recording of middle latency responses (MLR) in our routine. First we will obtain ABRs with a recording bandpass from 120 to 3,500 Hz, sweep time 20 ms, and a stimulus repetition rate of 20–30/s. The filter is then shifted to cover the range from 20 to 1,800 Hz, and with a sweep time of 50 ms the recordings are repeated at a stimulus rate of 10/s.

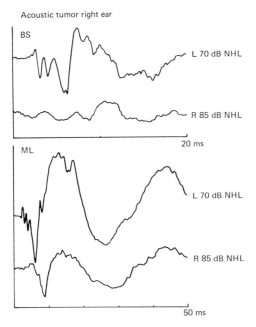

Acoustic tumor right ear

Fig. 4. Recordings from a patient with an acoustic neurinoma on the right side. The brainstem recordings are shown in the upper part of the figure and the MLRs in the lower part, where the high pass section of the recording filter is shifted from 120 to 20 Hz (3-dB points).

Figure 3 illustrates in a schematic way the configuration of the MLR as it appears with such a broad filter setting. Wave V of the ABR is very prominent as a deep, sharp vertex-positive peak, and the 3 main elements of the MLR – Na, Pa, and Nb – are also easily identifiable. We undertook a systematic evaluation of the MLR in a consecutive series of 33 neurinoma patients, where the PTA hearing impairment on the pathological ear was not greater than 80 dB. The most consistent waves proved to be Pa and Nb. The parameters that are indicated in figure 3 were submitted to a statistical analysis. The Pa latency in the normal ear response has a mean value of 23.5 ms with an SD of 2.5 ms. Ordinarily the MLR response that was elicited from the tumor ear was remarkably well preserved. The mean Pa latency here was 27.2 ms. This increase of latency was slightly more than the increase of wave V latency, and an analysis showed that the wave V-Pa difference is significant-

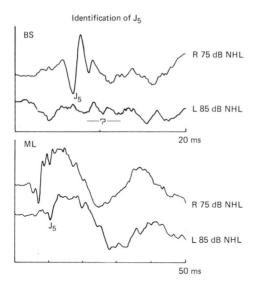

Fig. 5. Recordings from a patient with acoustic neurinoma on the left side. See text to figure 5.

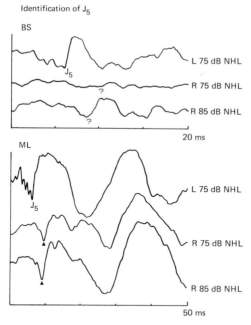

Fig. 6. Recordings from a patient with acoustic neurinoma on the right side. See text to figure 5.

ly longer on the tumor side $(0.01 < p < 0.02)$. The magnitude of the MLR on the other hand was much too variable to be of any help.

Figures 4–6 illustrate how well the so-called middle latency filter helps to identify wave V of the ABR. The ABRs for the normal and the pathological ear are shown in the upper part of the figures, and below that the MLRs. In all three cases the position or even the existence of wave V in the ABR from the tumor ear can be questioned. The MLRs clearly demonstrate that this is a matter only of recording technique and quite often our purpose would be served better by including more of the low frequencies in the recording filter if our specific aim is to evaluate wave V.

The techniques during these years develop so fast that these considerations may be valid only for a limited period of time. High resolution scanners will probably be very effective for the detection of even small tumors. When we use a screening approach by means of caloric testing, the ABR and tomography, it is because these procedures are cheap, easy to apply, and very effective. Our institution is in a 1,800-bed hospital, and we have 3 CT scanners. Cost-benefit evaluations, however, show that it would be far too expensive to use scanning as a first diagnostic approach. I am sure that high resolution scanners will be much more expensive and for some time to come a preliminary screening will be necessary, so that expensive or invasive procedures are reserved for the final diagnostic stages.

References

Terkildsen, K.; Osterhammel, O.; Thomsen, J.: The ABR and the MLR in patients with acoustic neuromas. Scand. Audiol. *13:* suppl., pp. 103–107 (1981).

Thomsen, J.; Nyboe, J.; Borum, P.; Tos, M.; Barfoed, C.: Acoustic neuromas. Archs Otolar. *107:* 601–607 (1981).

K. Terkildsen, MD, ENT Department, Rigshospitalet,
DK-2100 Copenhagen (Denmark)

Adv. Oto-Rhino-Laryng., vol. 29, pp. 68–71 (Karger, Basel 1983)

Audiological Assessment of Acoustic Tumours

Ian G. Taylor

Department of Audiology and Education of the Deaf, University of Manchester, Manchester, UK

The preoperative diagnosis of VIIIth nerve tumours is producing great interest at the present time because of the possibilities of effective surgical procedures to remove the tumours and preserve the facial nerve. However, the realities are often different in that patients are often seen with large tumours sometimes with long histories of increasing deafness.

This paper is concerned with reporting on 30 consecutive patients seen by the author's Department in collaboration with the Departments of Neurosurgery and Otolaryngology at Manchester. The audiometric procedures and findings together with the brain stem-evoked response are reported.

Patients and Procedure

All the cases were operated upon by *Dutton* and *Ramsden*, and in each case the confirmation of an acoustic tumour was made. The possibilities for audiometric procedure was sometimes limited by the critical state of the patients or where the degree of hearing loss in the affected ear was total. Of the 30 patients reported upon, 5 required shunt operation to reduce intercranial pressure before removal of the tumour was possible. 1 patient was too ill for any procedure apart from brain stem-evoked response testing. There were 2 patients with bilateral tumours. There were 10 patients whose deafness on the affected side was so severe that no audiometric procedures could be carried out on that side.

The audiometric tests carried out were those familiar to all: (1) Pure tone audiometry for air and bone conduction with masking where appropriate. (2) speech discrimination using monosyllabic words recorded on tape and played through headphones at the required loudness. Scores were plotted on a speech discrimination curve. (3) Tone decay. (4) Stapedial reflexes with special attention to asymmetry of 15 dB or greater. (5) Stapedial reflex decay. (6) Loudness recruitment using Hood's method.

For the brain stem-evoked response we place electrodes on the forehead (ground), vertex, left mastoid, right mastoid. The sound is delivered to each ear separately. Recordings are taken from the ipsilateral mastoid. Each ear is tested separately at a suprathreshold level. Each test is repeated to ensure test-retest reliability. Measurment of amplitude and latency of the observed waves are made and compared with our normal values. The stimulus used is a broad band click and filter cut-off points were set at $500 + 3,500$ Hz, *centred around 3 kHz*. 2,048 clicks are used at $25/s$ off 60-μs duration.

Results

Of the 30 patients examined: (1) 8 of the 20 patients examined using speech discrimination showed poorer discrimination than would have been expected from the pure tone audiogram. (2) 7/20 showed marked tone decay. (3) 8/18 showed reflex asymmetry where the differences between the two sides was 15 dB or greater. (4) 3/18 showed reflex decay. (5) 10/18 showed either partial or no recruitment. 2 patients gave one positive feature; 7 gave two; 2 gave three; 3 gave four, and no patients gave five positive features.

Results of the Brain Stem-Evoked Response Procedures

In particular we were interested in the latencies rather than the amplitudes. As our procedures allowed us to examine each ear separately we were interested both in the side of the tumour and in the contralateral side in the event of the effect of tumour being recorded on the 'good' side. As the origins of acoustic tumours is from the nerve fibre we could expect effects on the brain stem both on the side of the tumour as well as on the contralateral side depending whether the tumour was placed medially or laterally. The more medial the tumour the greater could be the effect on the contralateral side. These brain stem effects are not found in lesions of the cochlea and we would expect to find bilateral changes in space-occupying lesions of the posterior fossa.

We have developed our own coding system of the brain stem-evoked response results in order to make comparisons between and amongst patients. The findings of our results were as follows: In these patients the results on the contralateral side were more unexpected in that 8 of these showed a normal response whilst in one there was a reduced Vth nerve and in the other an absent V with the rest of the complex as normal. This is a finding which we associate with large tumours affecting the contralateral side. It will be appreciated that in patients who have a non-functional ear on subjective test procedures an absent or abnormal V wave is strong evidence of a large space-occupying lesion as distinct from a loss of hearing due to a peripheral loss.

Of the 11 cases who had good residual hearing on the affected side there were 5 who showed no consistent response despite the good pure tone audiometric results. There were 3 who had normal Ist and IInd waves but absent III, IV and V. There was 1 patient with a normal I but delay and reduced amplitudes in II and all others. There was 1 patient with a delay at III and onwards. There was 1 patient with a normal Ist but all others were absent. Of these 6 patients with various degrees of delay after the Ist wave, the responses on the contralateral ear were normal. In the 5 cases with inconsistent responses despite good pure tone audiometric thresholds (PTA), 3 had normal BSERs on the contralateral side. Of the other 2 both showed prolonged central conduction time. The inconsistent responses in these 5 cases is important to note in that the observation itself in the presence of good PTA is indicative of a retrocochlear lesion but not diagnostic. We have not found this BSER pattern in lesions of the chochlea.

We had 5 patients who required shunt operations in order to reduce intracranial pressure before removal of the tumour was possible. The results in these cases were as follows: 2 had no response in the ear of the tumour and the contralateral ear was normal; 1 had no response on the ear of the tumour and an absent Vth nerve on the contralateral side; 2 showed an inconsistent response pattern on the tumour side with, in 1 case, a prolonged central conduction time and, in the other, a normal BSER.

All 5 cases were found to have large tumours. There were 2 patients with bilateral tumours. In the 1st case, one side showed no response either on PTA or to BSER. On the second side there was a partial sensorineural loss with good speech discrimination. In the 2nd case there was no response either on PTA or the BSER. On the second side, despite only a partial loss on PTA, the speech discrimination was poorer than would be expected. In both cases despite good hearing on the second side there was no consistent response on the BSER.

In reviewing the whole of the BSER results, of the 25 patients examined by this procedure, 17 showed a positive result suggesting a retrocochlear lesion before operation, and 8 gave no positive results. Of the 17 patients with a positive BSER, 9 also showed other positive features during conventional audiometric test procedures with 8 who were not subjected to prolonged audiometry either because they were considered too unwell for further investigation, the diagnosis having been established, or the clinician did not request further investigation.

The final comment to be made concerning the BSER is that changes on the contralateral side can be observed following the removal of the tumour. We have followed up 17 of our cases. 11 were regarded as having normal BSER pre-operatively and 10 were so categorized post-operatively. 1 was found to have a prolonged conduction time post-operatively. This was in one of the patients with a large tumour who required a pre-removal shunt operation. 1 changed from a reduced V to normal. The 2nd with marginal delay returned to normal. 1 with a prolonged central conduction time returned to normal. 1 with an absent V remained with an absent V. The other with an absent V returned to normal. It is difficult to see a relationship between the changing patterns or otherwise of the BSER and conventional audiometry. As far as we can observe the non-tumour side functions normally whether or not we observe abnormalities of the BSER. A long-term follow-up study may reveal important facts.

In summary it is difficult to conclude by reference to data which can be treated for statistical significance. One of the most striking features is the great variability of each patient presenting with an acoustic tumour. Many are quite ill when first seen and allow for a limited audiological examination. No one test on conventional audiometry has been seen to be definitive in 100% of cases, which indicates the desirability of retaining a battery of the conventional audiometric test procedures. The BSER has proved to be a very valuable method of examination particularly when there is one non-functional ear and the ear on the contralateral side can be examined. It is most valuable in those patients who are too ill for conventional audiometry and in cases of bilateral tumours. However, we will require another occasion to discuss the value and indication of audiological procedures in comparison with CT scan and other investigations.

I.G. Taylor, MD, FRCP, Department of Audiology and Education of the Deaf, University of Manchester, Manchester M13 9PL (England)

Adv. Oto-Rhino-Laryng., vol. 29, pp. 72–88 (Karger, Basel 1983)

Audiological Assessment of Retrocochlear Lesions

Gunnar Lidén, Ulf Rosenhall

Department of Audiology and Otolaryngology, Sahlgren's Hospital, University of Göteborg, Sweden

The possibilities of diagnosing lesions affecting the 8th nerve, or the central auditory pathways in the brain stem or at higher levels have been improved considerably because of a tremendous development of new methods both in radiology and in audiology. The use of polytomography of the internal auditory meati, positive contrast cisternography and computerized tomography (CT scan) with or without contrast enhancement or in combination with pneumocisternography have significantly supplemented diagnoses based upon audiological measures.

The diagnosis of a neurological lesion in the auditory pathways requires a test battery. There is no single audiological test that provides the necessary information regarding location and extent of a lesion and of its disabling effects on the patient.

When a lesion affecting the auditory system is suspected, the first step is to perform pure tone and speech audiometry. Depending on these results Békésy audiometry, tone decay or alternate binaural loudness balance testing may be used. A further special audiologic test battery may appropriately include: (i) impedance audiometry; (ii) sound localization in freefield or lateralization tests (phase audiometry); (iii) distorted speech audiometry, and/or (iv) brain stem evoked response measurements (ABR).

The purpose of this paper is to report the clinical value of sound localization methods and to compare the results with those obtained with impedance audiometry and ABR in diagnosing neuroaudiological lesions.

The two last mentioned methods are well-known techniques and thus will not be described here [*Lidén* et al., 1981; *Rosenhall*, 1981]. Instead, we will focus on the use of the sound localization methods.

Several methods have been developed for the investigation of sound localization although two basic tests are presently in use: free-field tests or directional audiometry [*Jongkees and Groen*, 1946; *Nordlund*, 1963] and headphone tests with dichotic presentation called phase audiometry or lateralization test [*Matzker and Welker*, 1959; *Nilsson and Lidén*, 1976].

Basic Principles of Sound Localization

Directional hearing in the horizontal plane depends largely upon the acoustic differences between the stimulation of the right and the left ears. These interaural differences can be divided into time, phase, and intensity differences. This important auditory function has been studied in a great number of experiments [*Wightman and Firestone*, 1930; *von Békésy*, 1930; *Stevens and Newman*, 1936; *Nordlund*, 1962a, b; *Nordlund and Lidén*, 1963]. Directional hearing in the low frequency range is based on the ability of the individual to detect interaural phase and time differences [*Zwislocki and Feldman*, 1956]. The interaural intensity difference is of greatest importance for tones above 1,400 Hz. However, time difference becomes important in directional hearing of clicks, white noise or other complex sounds [*Christian and Röser*, 1957]. It has also been shown that directional hearing is better for low frequency pure tones [*Nordlund*, 1964].

The interaural time difference (ITD) as a function of azimuth (v) can be computed from the formula: ITD $= d/c$ and $d = a(v + \sin v)$, where d = the difference in distance which the sound has to travel to reach the ears, c = the velocity of sound (340 m/s), a = half the diametrical distance between ear orifices (0.085 m), and v is expressed as radian. Normally-hearing subjects tested with directional audiometry have a minimum audible angle of about 0.6 degrees [*Nilsson* et al., 1973]. The interaural time difference corresponding to this value is 5.2 μs, i.e. ITD $= 0.085 [0.6 \pi/180) + \sin 0.6]/340$.

There has been much conjecture as to the neural representation of interaural time and intensity differences. The model of binaural interaction proposed by *von Békésy* [1930] has ben further developed by *van*

Bergeijk [1962]. He suggested that time and intensity are mapped independent of each other in the accessory nuclei of the superior olive. Excitatory and inhibitory neural signals interact at the accessory nucleus neurons giving rise to a time-intensity trading function. Cells in both right and left accessory nuclei are innervated by excitatory fibers from the contralateral ear (cochlear nucleus) and inhibitory fibers from the ipsilateral ear. Ascending fibers from the two accessory nuclei transmit activity to a higher brain center where differences of interaural time and intensity are converted into differences in the number of cells excited. The quantitative difference in activity at this higher center forms a basis for lateralization judgements. In animal experimentation, *Hall* [1965] further elaborated on this theme by electrophysiological recordings from cells in the accessory nuclei sensitive to both interaural time and intensity difference. When the intensity of the stimuli to the two ears was held constant and the stimulus to the ipsilateral ear preceded the stimulus to the contralateral ear, the relative frequency of firing from these 'time-intensity trading' cells decreased. In a similar way the relative frequency of firing decreased when the stimulus at the ipsilateral ear was more intense than that at the contralateral ear and timing relationships were constant.

Jeffress [1975] expresses the situation somewhat differently by saying that there are at least two neural mechanism for sound localization. One is phaselocked to the stimulus with fibers that fire at a particular time in the sound cycle. The other is based upon the activity of fibers whose firing rate is determined by the level of the stimulus and is independent of the stimulus frequency.

It is, however, generally agreed that the superior olivary complex in the brain stem is the most peripheral (lowest) station in the ascending auditory pathways to receive information from both ears [*Neff* et al., 1975]. Since sound localization is based on time and intensity differences between the ears, disturbances of the neural impulses in one of the auditory nerves should show up in this measurement. Thus, lesions of the eighth nerve or the brain stem will render the center unable to carry out its function properly. The fusion of the signals coming from the periphery will not take place in the normal way and will give rise to disturbances in sound localization.

Different types of hearing deficits can influence directional hearing. Middle ear lesions often impair directional hearing. Lesions of the auditory nerve or the pontile region of the brain stem give noticeably abnormal directional hearing, whereas patients with temporal lobe lesions may have an entirely normal directional hearing. However, *Strominger and Neff* [1967] tested a patient who had a right hemispherectomy and found a small deficit in localizing in the horizontal plane when sounds are presented in the auditory field opposite the side of cortical damage. The auditory cortex also has an integrative function necessary for the perception of auditory space [*Masterson* et al., 1967].

Directional Audiometry

Free-field directional audiometry has been employed routinely in our laboratory for the last 20 years and has proved valuably in the diagnosis of retrocochlear lesions. Testing is performed in the following way. The horizontal location of a hidden mobile loudspeaker is varied in front of the test subject. Speaker positions are ordered on a scale so that the listener can respond with the scale number behind which he thinks the loudspeaker is located (fig. 1). Clinically, the test is now performed only with 500 Hz pure tone and low-pass filtered broad-band noise as stimuli. With the 500-Hz signal, the subject is free to move his head; the noise measurement is made under moveable and fixed head conditions. The sound intensity is set at a comfortable level for the patient but it must be sufficiently intense to be discerned by the more defective ear. The patient makes 20 judgements with the tone and 10 determinations with the noise. The results of the tests are then analyzed with regard to the mean of the differences (target mark) and the standard deviation of the judgement errors (target pattern). The mean of the minimum audible angle (MAA) for 100 normal-hearing subjects listening to a 500-Hz signal (20 judgements each) in an anechoic room with moveable head conditions was 0.6 degrees. Mean values outside the 99.0% confidence interval ± 8 degrees were only rated as pathological if the hearing threshold level differences for 500 Hz was not larger than 20 dB. The standard deviation for all 2,000 judgements of the 500-Hz tone was 2.3 degrees [*Nilsson* et al., 1973]. The borderline between normal and pathological values using 500 Hz and noise was set to 12 and 6 degrees, respectively [*Nordlund*, 1963]. Although we could make our borderline for 500 Hz more stringent we still maintain 12 degrees as the borderline for pathology for 500 Hz.

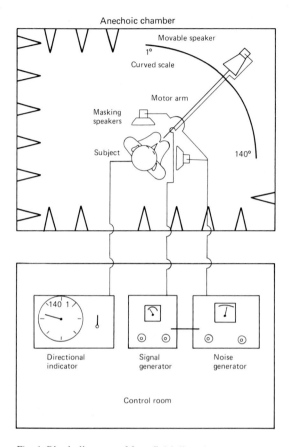

Fig. 1. Block diagram of free-field directional audiometry [*Nordlund, 1963*].

The ability to localize the 500-Hz tone mainly constitutes a measure of interaural phase differences. The interaural intensity difference is negligible [*Nordlund,* 1962a, b]. The ability to localize low pass filtered noise is a measure of interaural time differences. The discrimination of interaural intensity differences can be evaluated by investigating the ability to localize 2,000 and 4,000 Hz. However, these frequencies are found to be of minor diagnostic value and are excluded [*Lidén and Korsan-Bengtsen,* 1973].

Phase Audiometry

A second method of investigating time, phase and intensity differences separately involves the use of headphones with dichotic presentation. The subject listens to stimuli with variable differences in one of these parameters. A dichotically presented 500-Hz tone is perceived as an imaginary sound source moving inside the head of the listener depending on the interaural phase difference which is produced by an electronic phase shift unit. Normal listeners in a laboratory situation start to lateralize dichotically presented 500-Hz tone as soon as a difference in phase of 3–5 degrees is reached. A phase difference of one degree corresponds to a time difference of 5.56 μs ($= 1/360 \cdot 1/500$ s).

Matzker[1958a, b, 1966, 1967] and *Matzker and Welker*[1959] used a similar method with interrupted tonal signals as stimuli. Click artifacts at the onset of the signal were not eliminated. In spite of these clicks, frequency related differences in lateralization were found in patients with brain tumors. Interaural Δt's were adjusted until the patient lateralized the signal at intercranial midline. In cases with a unilateral cortical lesion, lateralizations judgements deviated to the side contralateral to the cortical lesion; in brain stem lesion to the side of the damage. *Matzker* thus concluded that his method made it possible to diagnose central hearing disorders and to draw certain conclusions regarding the site of the disease. *Groen* [1969], using similar equipment, stated, however, that Δt discrimination inability was only encountered in acoustic nerve disturbances. Unilateral disorders of the temporal lobe were not found to abolish Δt perception, although minimum Δt values might be increased slightly. This is in agreement with the findings of *Nordlund*[1964] but is in contrast to the opinion of *Matzker and Welker* [1959].

A disadvantage of free field directional audiometry is that it requires an anechoic room. In 1972, we developed phase audiometry in order to circumvent this problem. The equipment has been in the process of development and is now fully automated [*Nilsson* et al., 1973; *Nilsson and Lidén*, 1976; *Lidén* et al., 1977; *Lidén and Rosenhall*, 1982]. In one of these studies 60 normal hearing subjects were tested with phase audiometry in a clinical situation. The mean of the minimum interaural phase difference (IPD) expressed in degrees was 8.6° for the right ear and 8.6° for the left ear. The corresponding standard deviation were 3.3° and 3.6°. As borderline for possible pathology the mean

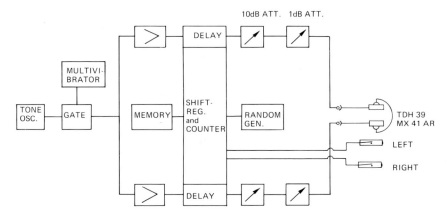

Fig. 2. Block diagram of the phase audiometer [*Nilsson and Lidén, 1976*].

of the IPD with three standard deviations was taken, i.e., 19 phase degrees. All of the 60 normal-hearing subjects studied had IPD below 17 degrees.

Figure 2 shows a block diagram of the phase audiometer. The oscillator generates a 500-Hz pure tone which can be presented binaurally with either continuous or pulsed tones (frequency 2.5 Hz, duration 200 μs, rise and decay time 40 μs) over headphones (THD 39, MX41AR). The maximum output, 110 dB SPL, can be adjusted by attenuators in 1-dB steps. The maximum phase shift, 90 degrees, produced by the electronic phase shift unit gives a perception of complete lateralization of the 500-Hz tone. The phase shift automatically diminishes in 2-degree decrements to 36 degrees and thereafter in 1 degree decrements. The generator for randomizing the presentations shifts the phase lag of the signal either to the right or to the left ear. At each test sequence, the tone used is first presented in the midline or center of the head without phase lag, and then with phase lag. The patient administers the test himself, and is able to record the ear in which the tone was heard.

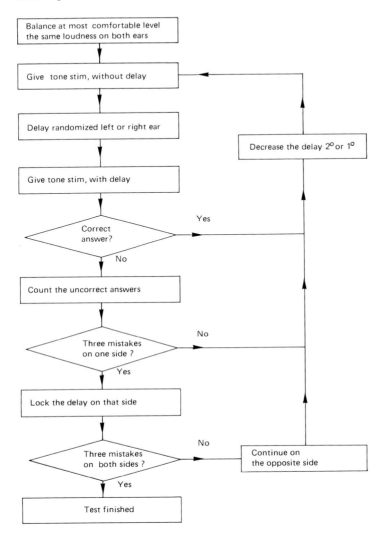

Fig. 3. Flow diagram of the function of the phase audiometer [*Nilsson and Lidén,* 1976].

Procedure

The 500-Hz tone is presented binaurally with headphones. The intensity at each ear is individually adjusted to yield a midline perception with a zero phase difference at a comfortable loudness level. Thus, we compensate for a threshold difference between the two ears. This has to be done carefully because a difference in levels of only 0.7 dB be-

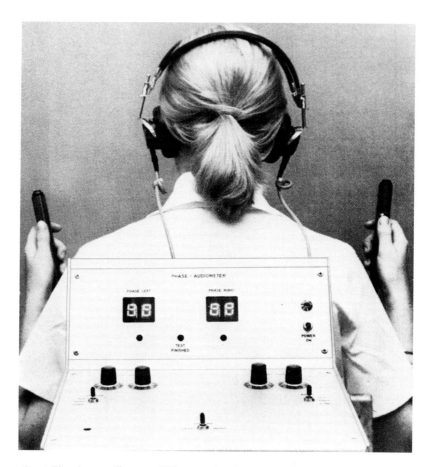

Fig. 4. The phase audiometer [*Nilsson and Lidén,* 1976].

tween the ears gives rise to a just noticeable shift of the sound image from midline [*Mills,* 1972]. It is important to note that the test cannot be carried out in patients with asymmetrical hearing losses of such degree that a midline impression of equal loudness cannot be achieved. The test starts by adjusting the audiometer on position automatic. One of the test channels will produce a maximum phase lag of 90 degrees. The patient hears the tone in his opposite ear and records this accordingly. The phase lag is then reduced to zero and the patient hears the tone in the midline position. Thereafter the phase shift is decreased by 2 degrees, i.e. a tone with a phase shift of 88 degrees is presented to one of the ears. This phase shift is presented randomly between ears to minimize preselection by the patient. As long as the subject responds correctly, the phase shift diminishes automatically on successive trials as previously described. A counter samples incorrect responses, and terminates the test when three errors have occurred on each side. A flow diagram of

Table I. Results of phase audiometry in normal and hearing-impaired subjects

Type	Minimum interaural phase difference in degrees: normal borderline 19°			
	n	mean	SD	percent abnormal
Normal	60	8.6	3.3	0
Cochlear	16	14.8	4.4	6
Cerebellopontine angle tumors	40	58	30	78
Brain stem tumors	14	49	29	71
Cerebellar tumors	9	29	16	56
Vascular brain stem lesions	26	47	26	80
Supratentorial lesions	22	18	11	14

the function of the phase audiometer is given in figure 3. The examiner can follow the gradually diminishing phase shift for both ears on a digital display (fig. 4). By the step-wise decrease in phase shift, the patients tested are able to gain experience in performing the test, so that testing time often averages 10 min. While efficiency in performing the test may increase with practice the final result does not change [*Nilsson and Lidén,* 1976]. When the result of the test is pathological the whole test is repeated three times.

Material

The patient material consists of 41 cerebellopontine angle tumors, 14 brain stem tu-mors, 9 cerebellar tumors, 26 vascular brain stem lesions and 22 supratentorial lesions. The cases with vascular brain stem lesions were diagnosed with neurological, ophthal-moneurological and sometimes with neuroradiological tests (CT scan and vertebral an-giography). In all cases of vascular brain stem lesions the auditory pathways in the brain stem were involved, as shown by the different audiological tests (impedance audiometry, distorted speech audiometry, tone decay test, sound localization tests and ABR).

In addition, 22 cases of supratentorial lesions were studied with sound localization tests. 11 of these cases had brain tumors, 3 had vascular cerebral lesions, 2 severe concus-sion of the brain, and 6 had other cerebral lesions such as viral encephalitis with focal neurological signs. For comparison, 16 subjects with cochlear hearing loss and 60 with normal hearing were included.

Table II. Results of free-field directional audiometry in normal and hearing-impaired subjects

Type	n	Means of standard deviations in degrees			
		500 Hz normal limits SD 12	LP noise MH normal limits SD 6	LP noise FH normal limits SD 6	percent abnormal
Normal	51	4.6	2.0	2.7	0
Cochlear	22	6.1	2.9	3.4	0
Cerebellopontine angle tumors	28	15.0	12.1	10.0	75
Brain stem tumors	4	11.6	12.0	12.3	100
Cerebellar tumors	4	9.9	7.0	6.7	50
Vascular brain stem lesions	24	11.5	8.8	6.6	42
Supratentorial lesions	15	5.8	3.4	3.4	7

MH = Moveable head; FH = fixed head; LP = low pass.

Results

Phase and Directional Audiometry

Generally speaking, automatic phase audiometry is easy to perform. Even bedridden patients can perform the test. The decision to terminate the test after three incorrect responses on each side as a final threshold value was partially based on the finding that normal-hearing subjects were capable of reaching threshold levels without three errors. The automatic locking of the phase shift after three mistakes also makes threshold determination easier. In this way, the effect of excessive guessing of the final threshold values is avoided.

The results of phase audiometry and free field directional audiometry are given in tables I and II. Values for normal-hearing subjects as well as for 16 persons with cochlear losses are included for comparison. Most patients with cochlear or supratentorial lesions performed well on the tests.

40 patients with cerebellopontine angle tumors were tested with phase audiometry and 28 with directional audiometry. 78% of the tested subjects were pathological using phase audiometry and 75% using

Table III. Results of impedance audiometry

Type	n	Strapedius reflex threshold abnormal		n	Strapedius reflex decay abnormal %
		n	%		
Cerebellopontine angle tumors	41	35	85	12	50
Brain stem tumors	12	9	75	7	14
Cerebellar tumors	9	6	67	4	25
Vascular brain stem lesions	26	13	50		

directional audiometry. The cases with brain stem tumors gave abnormal results with phase audiometry in 71%. With directional audiometry all patients showed pathological results. The subjects with cerebellar tumors gave about 50% abnormal values with both sound localization methods. Patients with vascular brain stem lesions affecting the auditory pathways gave 80% abnormal values with phase audiometry but only 42% were pathological according to directional audiometry. Of the 22 subjects with supratentorial lesions 3 (14%) had abnormal values with phase audiometry and only one with directional audiometry.

As can be seen from tables I and II, there is generally a good correlation between phase and directional audiometry although there are fewer patients investigated with the last-mentioned method. The only exception is brain stem lesions in which the two methods gave contradictory results.

Impedance Audiometry

In the 41 cases of cerebellopontine angle tumors (acoustic neuromas and other cerebellopontine angle tumors) impedance audiometry showed signs of retrocochlear lesion in 35 cases (85%) (table III). These signs are elevated reflex thresholds (16 cases) or absent reflexes (19 cases) and/or pathological stapedius reflex decay ('half-life' of reflex response amplitude below 5 s on stimulation with 500 and 1,000 Hz tones) [*Anderson* et al., 1969]. The reflex decay test was performed in 12 cases, and was found to be pathological only in 6 cases which also had pathological elevated reflex thresholds. The cases with brain stem and cerebellar tumors gave pathological results in 75 and 67%, respectively.

Table IV. Results of brain stem evoked response in cerebellopontine, brain stem and cerebellar tumors

Type	N	A	B	C	D	Abnormal, %
Cerebellopontine angle tumors	21	1	6	14		100
Brain stem tumors	6		3	3		100
Cerebellar tumors	6		1	3	2	100

A = No response; B = later ABR components missing; C = increased wave V latency; D = decreased amplitudes of waves IV and/or V (borderline pathology).

The decay tests were abnormal in 14 and 25%. The vascular brain stem lesions gave 50% abnormal impedance audiometry results.

Brain Stem Evoked Response Measurements

ABR was obtained on 21 cases with cerebellopontine angle tumors. All were pathological. In 6 cases the later ABR components were missing and 14 cases had prolonged wave-V latency. The brain stem and the cerebellar tumors were all pathological (table IV).

Comparison between the Special Tests

Table V and figure 5 show the results of the sound localization tests, impedance audiometry and ABR. ABR audiometry showed to be superior to all tests used. The sound localization tests and impedance audiometry indicated abnormal results in about 80% of the cases with cerebellopontine angle tumors. Phase audiometry was also a good indication of pathology in brain stem lesions.

Discussion

Earlier investigations with young adult psychoacoustically trained test subjects in laboratory situations have indicated that for 500 Hz the minimum interaural time difference in dichotic presentations which produces an impression of deviation from the midline is approximately 17 μs (3 phase degrees) [*Klumpp and Eady*, 1956]. In a free-field situation, an interaural time difference of 17 μs will correspond to a MAA difference of about 2 degrees. The average MAA in directional audio-

Table V. Results of sound localization tests, impedance audiometry and brain stem evoked response measurements in 112 patients with cerebellopontine, brain stem and cerebellar tumors, vascular brain stem lesions and supratentorial lesions

Type	Phase audiometry		Directional audiometry		Impedance audiometry		Brain stem evoked responses	
	n	% ab-normal	n	% ab-normal	n	% ab-normal	n	% ab-normal
Cerebellopontine angle tumors	40	78	28	75	41	85	21	100
Brain stem tumors	14	71	4	100	12	75	6	100
Cerebellar tumors	9	56	4	50	9	67	6	100
Vascular brain stem lesions	26	80	24	42	26	50	–	–
Supratentorial lesions	22	14	15	7	–	–	–	–

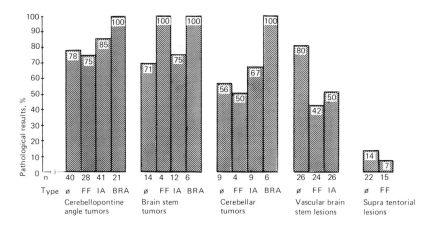

ø Phase audiometry
FF Free field directional audiometry
IA Impedance audiometry
BRA Brain stem audiometry

Fig. 5. Results of phase and directional audiometry in comparison with impedance audiometry and brain stem evoked response measurements in 112 patients with retrocochlear, brain stem, cerebellar and supratentorial lesions.

metry is 1 degree, thus making it more sensitive than phase audiometry. Interaural phase difference thresholds determined with phase audiometry on normal-hearing young subjects in a clinical situation are higher (8.6°). One explanation for this fact may be that the test automatically terminates after three errors at each ear.

In the free-field sound localization test, the minimum detectable angle difference is based on time and/or intensity differences between the ears. By turning the head toward the sound source, the interaural differences are equalized. In this way, we sharpen our ability to localize sounds. This advantage is of course lost in phase audiometry. From the physical point of view, phase audiometry could be compared to free-field localization with the head fixed. The performance difference in the vascular brain stem lesions between phase and directional audiometry (table I, II) probably reflects the elimination of head movement and the restriction of performance to the use of one cue (phase difference). All neurophysiological models agree that with this reduction the task must be somewhat more difficult and performance more susceptible to disruption by a restricted lesion.

Phase audiometry is thus more sensitive for identifying vascular brain stem lesions than free field localization and this test profile can be used in clinical practice. In the three tumor groups, however, such a difference is not obvious.

The disadvantage with phase audiometry is that the subject localizes the sound source in his head or in its close proximity. This implies, as *Nordlund* [1964] has already pointed out, that the same degree of accuracy may not be obtained as in the more physiological situation; i.e., when sound is presented in a free-field. Moreover, it can also be questioned whether the same response is being investigated, since in one situation the sound is seemingly located inside the head whereas in the other instance the sound is located in the room. Electrophysiological data, however, do suggest that neural mechanisms, at least at the brain stem level, are similar if not identical.

Impedance audiometry is a very good indicator of acoustic neuromas and other cerebellopontine angle tumors. When a lesion is located higher up in the brain stem or in the cerebellum impedance audiometry is less reliable.

Brain stem evoked response measurements are more time consuming than the other methods but have up to now given the most paramount results.

Conclusion

From our clinical experiences we can conclude the following: (i) In patients with neuroaudiological symptoms a test battery including ABR, sound localization tests and impedance audiometry should be used. (ii) ABR seems to be the most reliable indicator of retrocochlear and brain stem lesions. (iii) Phase audiometry is a useful clinical test, and provides an alternative to free field directional audiometry in testing patients for possible retrocochlear and brain stem lesions.

References

Anderson, H.; Barr, B.; Wedenberg, E.: Intra-aural reflexes in retrocochlear lesions; in Hamberger, Wersäll Nobelsymposium 10: Disorders of the skull base region, p. 49 (Almqvist-Wiksell, Stockholm 1969).

Békésy, G. von: Zur Theorie des Hörens. Physiol. Z. *31:* 824 (1930).

Bergeijk, W. van: Variation on a theme of Békésy. A model of binaural interaction. J. acoust. Soc. Am. *34:* 1431 (1962).

Christian, W.; Röser, D.: Ein Beitrag zum Richtungshören. Z. Lar. Rhinol. Otol. *36:* 431 (1957).

Groen, J.: Diagnostic value of lateralization ability for dichotic time differences. Acta oto-lar. *67:* 326 (1969).

Hall, J.L.: Binaural interaction in the accessory superior-olivary nucleus of the cat. J. acoust. Soc. Am. *37:* 814 (1965).

Jeffress, L.A.: Localization of sound; in Keidel, Neff, Handbook of sensory physiology (Springer, Berlin 1975).

Jongkees, L.; Groen, J.: On directional hearing. J. Lar. Otol. *61:* 494 (1946).

Klumpp, R.; Eady, H.: Some measurements of interaural time-difference thresholds. J. acoust. Soc. Am. *28:* 859 (1956).

Lidén, G.; Björkman, G.; Renvall, U.: Impedance audiometry for diagnosing and screening middle ear lesions; in Penha, Noronka Pizarro, Proc. 4th Int. Symp. Acoustic Impedance Measurements, University of Lisboa, 1981.

Lidén, G.; Korsan-Bengtsen, M.: Audiometric manifestations of retrocochlear lesions. Adv. Oto-Rhino-Laryng., vol. 20, p. 271 (Karger, Basel 1973).

Lidén, G.; Nilsson, E.; Nilsson, R.: Sound localization with phase audiometry. Proc. of XI Wld Congr. Otorhinolaryngology, Buenos Aires 1977; part II, p. 681.

Lidén, G.; Rosenhall, U.: New developments in diagnostic auditory-neurological problems; in Paparella, Meyerhoff, Sensorineural hearing loss, vertigo and tinnitus (Williams & Wilkins, Baltimore 1981).

Masterson, B.; Jane, J.; Diamond, L.: Role of brain stem auditory structures in sound localization. J. Neurophysiol. *30:* 341 (1967).

Matzker, J.: Modell der synaptischen Schaltung in den Hirnstammkernen der Hörbahn. Z. Lar. Rhinol. Otol. *37:* 167 (1958a).

Matzker, J.: Versuch einer Erklärung des Richtungshörens auf Grund feinster Zeitunterschiedsregistrierungen. Acta oto-lar. *49:* 483 (1958b).

Matzker, J.: Die Kompensation seitenverschiedener Hörstörungen bei der Prüfung des Richtungshörens mit elektrisch erzeugten Laufzeitdifferenzen. Z. Lar. Rhinol. Otol. *45:* 331 (1966).

Matzker, J.: Der 'binaurale Click-Test' zur Diagnose zerebraler Hörstörungen. Z. Lar. Rhinol. Otol. *46:* 101 (1967).

Matzker, J.; Welker, H.: Die Prüfung des Richtungshörens zum Nachweis und zur topischen Diagnostik von Hirnerkrankungen. Z. Lar. Rhinol. Otol. *38:* 277 (1959).

Mills, W.: Auditory localization; in Tobias, Foundations of modern auditory theory, vol. II (Academic Press, New York 1972).

Neff, W.D; Diamond, I.T.; Casseday, J.H.: Behavioral studies of auditory discrimination. Central nervous system: in Keidel, Neff, Handbook of sensory physiology, vol. V/2, p. 307 (Springer, Berlin 1975).

Nilsson, R.; Lidén, G.: Sound localization with phase audiometry. Acta oto-lar. *81:* 291 (1976).

Nilsson, R.; Lidén, G.; Rosén, M.; Zöller, M.: Directional hearing, three different testmethods. Scand. Audiol. *2:* 125 (1973).

Nordlund, B.: Physical factors in angular localization. Acta oto-lar. *54:* 75 (1962a).

Nordlund, B.: Angular localization. Acta oto-lar. *55:* 405 (1962b).

Nordlund, B.: Studies of stereophonic hearing; thesis Göteborg (1963).

Nordlund, B.: Directional audiometry. Acta oto-lar. *57:* 1 (1964).

Nordlund, B.; Lidén, G.: An artificial head. Acta oto-lar. *56:* 493 (1963).

Rosenhall, U.: Brain stem electrical responses in cerebello-pontine angle tumours. J. Lar. Otol. *95:* 931 (1981).

Stevens, S.; Newman, E.: The localization of actual sources of sound. Am. J. Psychol. *48:* 297 (1936).

Strominger, N.; Neff, W.: Sound localization in temporal lobe operated patients. (Abstract). Anat. Rec. (1967): cited in Keidel, Neff, Handbook of sensory physiology, vol. V/2, p. 355 (Springer, Berlin 1975).

Wightman, E.; Firestone, F.: Binaural localization of pure tones. J. acoust. Soc. Am. *2:* 271 (1930).

Zwislocki, J.; Feldman, R.S.: Just noticeable differences in dichotic phase. J. acoust. Soc. Am. *28:* 860 (1956).

G. Lidén, MD, Department of Audiology and Otolaryngology, Sahlgren's Hospital, University of Göteborg, S-41345 Göteborg (Sweden)

Adv. Oto-Rhino-Laryng., vol. 29, pp. 89–101 (Karger, Basel 1983)

Clinical Investigation of the Efferent Inhibition of the Vestibular Function

Erik Fluur

Department of Otolaryngology, Södersjukhuset, Stockholm, Sweden

All those working with otoneurology know that there are often patients in whom none of the traditional nystagmus parameters, such as threshold, latency time, amplitude, duration or speed of the slow phase give any tenable information. There are patients with such an enormous dysrhythmia that all evaluations are impossible. There are also persons who display a total inhibition during stimulation, but are getting a very adequate nystagmus as soon as the stimulus has ceased. Such oscillations in the nystagmus picture cannot be due to an organic damage to the peripheral labyrinth but must have its cause in a functional variation in the vestibular afferent impulse pattern. The question is at what level should this modulation take place, peripherally or centrally. We know today from many publications that the signals from the labyrinth can be modulated by inhibition or facilitation of efferent impulses from the central nervous system. But we also know that many central factors, for instance wakefulness, oculomotor activation and psychological disturbances have an influence on the nystagmus. Thus, the entire reaction will be changed when we stimulate the patient and all the old and well-known nystagmus parameters will no longer be as reliable as we have believed. As a consequence of this we have abandoned the old principle to look at different parameters in favor of looking at the nystagmus pattern more from an integrated or holistic point of view. In this way we think we have found a clinical method to investigate the entire physiological activity during stimulation including the efferent modulation. We wanted to put this modulation into a wider context and elucidate what function it has in the vestibular reaction as a whole. We have also asked if the efferent inhibition is a defence me-

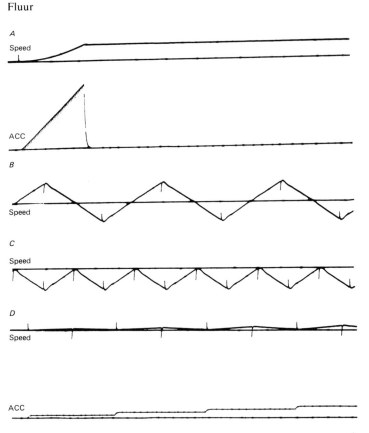

Fig. 1. *A* Symbol of constant increasing accerelation. *B* Symbol of bidirectional triangular oscillation. *C* Symbol of unidirection triangular oscillation. *D* Symbol stepwise increasing acceleration.

chanism against too strong vestibular stimuli just like the stapedic reflex against strong sounds or if it has a continuously modulating influence on the input from the labyrinth just like the pupillary reflex against light.

In order to answer the above-mentioned questions we have studied 30 normal persons and about 4,000 otoneurological patients with a rotation test battery according to certain computerized test programs (fig. 1). To ascertain whether the efferent inhibition has a threshold at a certain stimulation level we have used a constantly increasing acceleration by which the cupula is performing a sliding movement across the surface of the crista giving a constantly increasing deflexion of the sen-

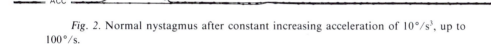

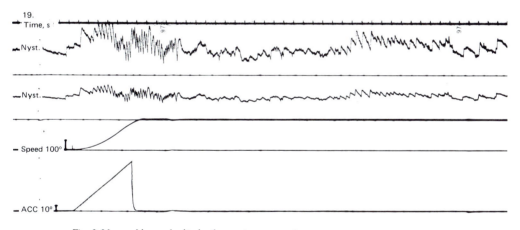

Fig. 2. Normal nystagmus after constant increasing acceleration of $10°/s^3$, up to $100°/s$.

Fig. 3. Normal irregularity in the nystagmus pattern.

sory hairs. We have used two different tests, one slow with an acceleration increase of $0.1°/s$ with a final acceleration of $4°/s^2$ and another fast with $10°/s$ and a final acceleration of $50°/s^2$. The slow program is used primarily in order to study latency times and hypo- and hyperreflexia, the fast for investigation of inhibition.

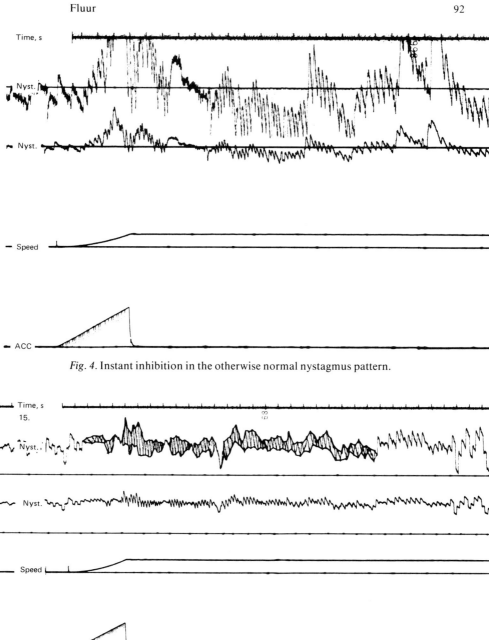

Fig. 4. Instant inhibition in the otherwise normal nystagmus pattern.

Fig. 5. Irregular nystagmus pattern in a dizzy patient. The upper nystagmus curve is filled in order to accentuate the modulation.

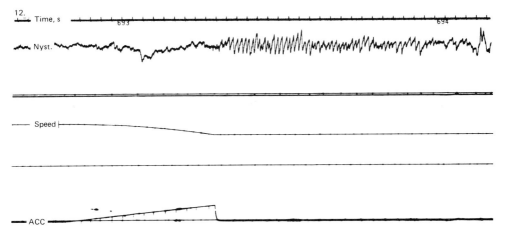

Fig. 6. Total inhibition during the acceleration, but otherwise normal reaction.

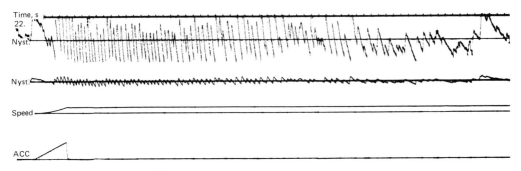

Fig. 7. Nystagmus picture in a hyperreflexive patient.

The experiments with 30 normal persons did not show any inhibition at a certain strength of stimulation at least not on stimuli up to $50°/s^2$. On the other hand, it turned out that different persons react very differently to the same stimulus. Normally the nystagmus reaches a maximum intensity and disappears slowly at a constant speed (fig. 2). In many persons there is a normal response during weak stimuli but at $50°/s^2$ the nystagmus becomes irregular, the frequency increases rapidly and the amplitude decreases, sometimes almost down to total inhibition. When the nystagmus intensity decreases the reaction slowly returns again and disappears in a normal way (fig. 3). In other persons

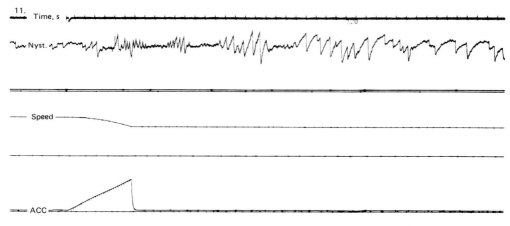

Fig. 8. Repeated inhibition periods in a hyperreflexive patient.

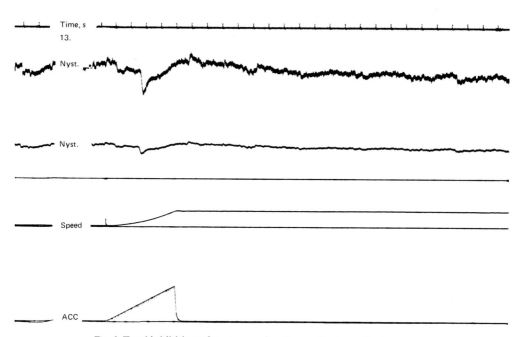

Fig. 9. Total inhibition of nystagmus in a hyporeflexive patient.

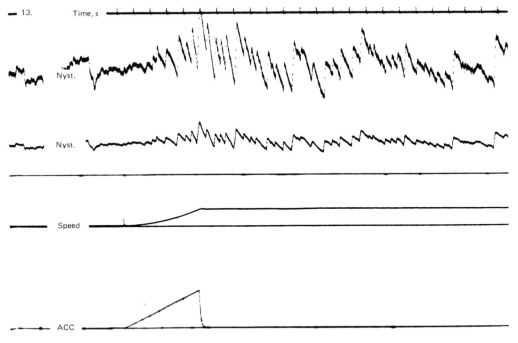

Fig. 10. The nystagmus reaction in the same patient as figure 12, but during simultaneous counting backwards.

the inhibition comes instantaneously with a duration of 1–2 s followed by a sudden reappearance of nystagmus (fig. 4).

There are many dizzy patients who react the same way as normal persons but more intensively. Certain patients have a very irregular nystagmus but no total inhibition (fig. 5). Others have a total inhibition during the acceleration but normal response as soon as the stimulus has changed into constant speed (fig. 6).

Of special interest are investigations made on hyperreflexive patients. Here the latency time is much shorter, the nystagmus more intensive and the duration much longer than in normal persons. The nystagmus panorama is remarkably regular without modulations. The patients often have subjective discomfort, which makes the investigation difficult (fig. 7). In many of these patients we have found something which never happens in normal persons, namely several short periods of total sudden inhibition during 1–10 s. The nystagmus disappears momentarily after a fast phase, and the eyes are kept completely still in

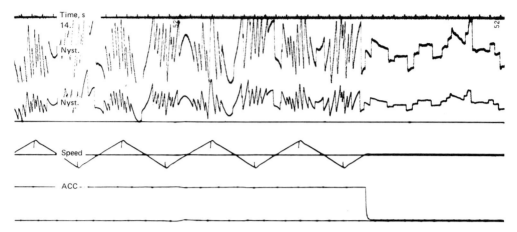

Fig. 11. Normal nystagmus reaction during bidirectional oscillation.

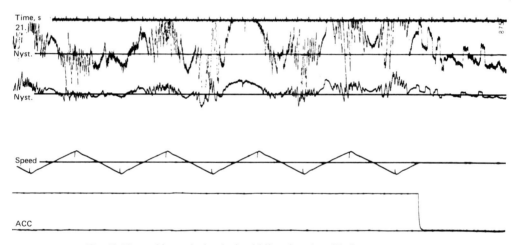

Fig. 12. Normal irregularity during bidirectional oscillation.

the midline or move slowly in an undefinable direction. After this the nystagmus reappears suddenly with unchanged frequency and rapidly increasing amplitude (fig. 8). These periods of inhibition may be isolated or be repeated during the same stimulation. They are in no way random and can be reproduced several times.

Sometimes, but more rarely, we see the opposite category of patients, those who are hyporeflexive, who do not react either to caloric or rotatory stimulation during the first investigation (fig. 9), but who

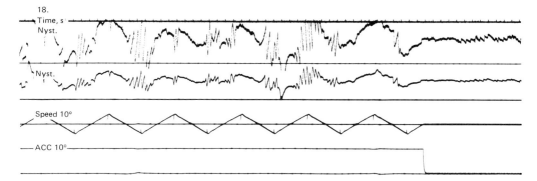

Fig. 13. Inhibition periods during oscillation of a dizzy patient, getting nystagmus after finishing the oscillation.

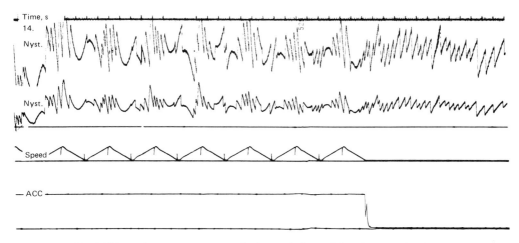

Fig. 14. Normal nystagmus pattern during and after unidirectional oscillation.

react very distinctly if they simultaneously count loudly from 300 every or every second number backwards (fig. 10).

Another way of studying the influence of the central nervous system on the vestibular reactions is to oscillate the patient (fig. 1b). They are exposed ten times to a triangular oscillation with $60°/s^2$ up to $120°/s$. The cupula is then forced from one stationary position to another. The normal person is thus getting a regular nystagmus alternating to the right or to the left (fig. 11). In some persons a certain irregu-

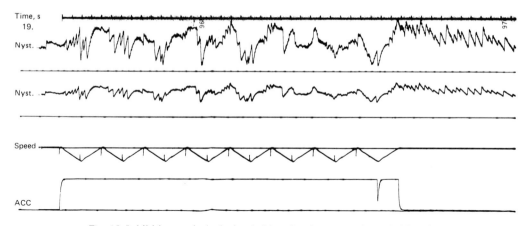

Fig. 15. Inhibition periods during habituation but normal posthabituation nystagmus in the opposite direction.

larity with smaller inhibitions is found, but the normal nystagmus always returns again (fig. 12). When the oscillation has finished the person has been stimulated equally in both directions and therefore no postrotatory nystagmus is obtained. The oscillation of patients showed that many had periods of more or less total inhibition during the oscillation, sometimes in one nystagmus direction, sometimes in both. But after a few oscillations the nystagmus returns with the same intensity as before. When the oscillation has finished many patients with a disturbed balance between the right and left side get a nystagmus towards the side with the higher activity (fig. 13).

An additional way of studying the efferent influence on vestibular stimuli is to habituate the labyrinths one by one (fig. 1c). This is done by oscillating the patient in such a way that he gets a nystagmus in one direction only. However, at a certain point, nystagmus beats grow in the opposite direction. The threshold of the first beat is about $10°/s^2$. After finishing the oscillation, the person gets a postrotatory nystagmus, beating in the opposite direction to the perrotatory as a sign of habituation (fig. 14). In most patients the posthabituation nystagmus in the opposite direction is equal in both sides, but sometimes large differences can be seen. In these cases the threshold for the first nystagmus beat in the opposite direction is also different. Patients with hyperreflexia display short lively periods of inhibition in the primary nystagmus pattern, but the posthabituation nystagmus is not changed com-

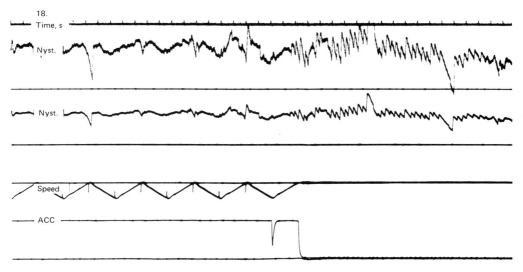

Fig. 16. Total inhibition during habituation but nevertheless normal posthabituation nystagmus in the opposite direction.

pared with normal persons (fig. 15). Other patients have a total inhibition during the whole stimulation but nevertheless get a normal postrotatory nystagmus in the opposite direction after the habituation (fig. 16).

By these results we have ascertained that the efferent inhibition does not function as the stapedic reflex but modulates the nystagmus as a kind of defence mechanism against too intensive stimuli ad modum the pupillary reflex. The fact that normal persons react sometimes with inhibition of nystagmus shows that this is a normal reaction, which is activated when the person experiences the stimulus as disagreable.

The investigation has shown that there are two main groups of pathological reactions with every variation in between, one hyperreflexive group with excessively intensive nystagmus even at weak stimuli, and one hyporeflexive group where the patient does not react at all to normal stimuli, but gets a normal response if he simultaneously counts loudly backwards. The investigation has also shown that there seems to be two different types of inhibition, one fast, appearing during intensive reactions and having a short duration, short time constant (STC), high gain and high reaction readiness, and another type, which is slow and habituating and coming first after iterated stimuli and having a long duration, long time constant (LTC), low initial gain and low reaction readiness.

One can ask if these two reaction patterns can be explained by a difference in efferent output to the labyrinths or if higher centers are involved. It appears as if the efferent fibers normally are more or less spontaneously active. This means that the normal afferent labyrinthine input is always under a certain negative feedback from the opposite side and from different higher centers. However, as we have seen in the introduction there is also a facilitatory positive feedback to the labyrinth. All these feedbacks together provoke what we call a normal vestibular response when we stimulate the semicircular canals. If this negative feedback is missing or the facilitation is increased the reaction readiness will be enhanced and the patient gets a hyperreflexia when stimulated. If, on the other hand, the patient has an elevated negative feedback level or a missing facilitation, he will be hyporeflexive and not react to normal stimuli.

However, this explanation does not seem to fit in with the present results. As mentioned earlier the inhibition of nystagmus is a normal reaction to disagreable stimuli. It has been shown that hyperreflexive patients have more extensive inhibitions than normal persons. The question is whether that can be considered as pathological. This does not seem to be the case, but merely a result of an increased activity level which the patient experiences as disagreeable and therefore activates his STC inhibitions.

There are certain findings in the present investigation which speak in favor of a central genesis. This is supported by the findings that inhibition often grows via a sudden initial increase in frequency, despite the fact that the stimulus has finished. One possibility is an increasing input from higher centers to the nystagmogenic centers, finally leading to a clonic contraction of the eye muscles and by this a total inhibition of nystagmus. Another possibility is that the macronystagmus disappears suddenly and the micronystagmus remains for a few seconds in some persons but not in others, because it also happens that the nystagmus simply disappears without any increase in frequency.

Another supporting finding is the fact that hyporeflexive patients get a normal reaction if, simultaneously with the stimulus, they are asked to count loudly backwards. Whether this is an effect of arousal via reticular formation or of a disinhibition of the cerebellar nodulus or flocculus is difficult to say.

Still another factor supporting this idea is the fact that many hyperreflexive patients during oscillation for monolabyrinthine habituation have a total inhibition during the oscillation but are nevertheless displaying a normal postrotatory nystagmus in the opposite direction after habituation. If the perrotatory inhibition were elicited in the peripheral labyrinth there would have been a more or less total cancellation of all input from the semicircular canals and thus no triggering of the cerebellar centers, responsible for habituation, would have been possible.

Therefore, our conclusion is that this STC or – if you want – emergency inhibition seems to take place in centers higher up than the vestibular organs. A conceivable site could be the reticular formation. Here we have a large integrating center, from which wakefulness, nystagmus and possibly even other functions can be modulated and – as we have seen here – also totally inhibited without the participation of the labyrinths. The fact that psychological circumstances can affect the amount of modulation also indicates that higher centers can be involved.

Concerning the LTC inhibitions the investigation has shown that, following the habituating oscillation, the patient gets postrotatory nystagmus in the opposite direction to the perrotatory, even if there is a complete inhibition of nystagmus during the oscillations. This indicates that there is continuous input from the labyrinths during the lack of measurable nystagmus, which stimulates the Purkinje cells of the cerebellar nuclei, giving an inhibition of one labyrinth and a facilitation of the other. This also indicates that STC and LTC are working more or less independently of each other, which means that we have to accept a second inhibitory system. The target for this inhibition seems to be the peripheral labyrinths. This is in agreement with many observations that this modulation is triggered directly from the labyrinth itself through a feedback via the cerebellum back to the labyrinth.

The conclusion of this investigation is that it indicates two different inhibition systems, one central and one peripheral, which can both be subjected to clinical investigation and which provide us with important information both about the way the central nervous system modulates the peripheral signals and also about the cause of many cases of so-called vestibular vertigo.

Erik Fluur, MD, Department of Otolaryngology, Södersjukhuset,
S-100 64 Stockholm 38 (Sweden)

Adv. Oto-Rhino-Laryng., vol. 29, pp. 102–110 (Karger, Basel 1983)

Visual Suppression Test

Setsuko Takemori

Neurotology, Toranomon Hospital, Tokyo, Japan

Introduction

Visual suppression is one method to examine the function of visual fixation. Visual fixation is very important for the maintenance of equilibrium. It is well-known that the vestibular nystagmus is inhibited by visual fixation [4, 6]. Frenzel glasses are very widely used to evoke nystagmus by eliminating visual fixation in the clinic [2].

Recently, visual fixation was examined by measuring and comparing the slow-phase velocity of caloric nystagmus in darkness and in light, and this method is called visual suppression [7, 11]. Visual suppression in various kinds of diseases was studied to clarify the mechanisms of visual fixation.

Methods

Eye movements were recorded by electronystagmography (ENG) using silver-plate electrodes. The time constant for eye movement recordings was 3 s and for eye velocity recordings 0.03 s. Eye movements were differentiated to obtain velocity measures and clipped to display the slow-phase velocity. An upward pen deflection indicated eye movements to the right.

Subjects lay on a bed with their heads raised 30° during the examination at the clinic. The examiner's index finger was held 50 cm above the subject and it was the point used to fix their eyes on.

20 ml of water at 5 °C was used to irrigate the external auditory canal during a 20-second light period with the eyes open and covered. The room lights were turned off for 30–45 s. During this period, the slow-phase velocity of caloric nystagmus reached a maximum. The lights were then turned on for 10 s with the eyes open and fixed on a target.

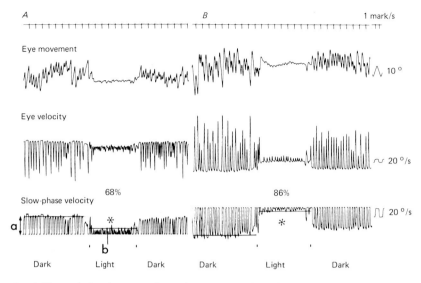

Fig. 1. Normal visual suppression. Visual suppression of a normal subject is shown. *A* Caloric nystagmus to the left. *B* Caloric nystagmus to the right. The asterisks show visual suppression. The eye movement recordings are the DC recordings.

This caused an immediate suppression of the slow-phase velocity of caloric nystagmus. At the end of this period, the room lights were turned off again and the eyes were covered until the end of caloric nystagmus.

The mean slow-phase velocity of the maximum responses of caloric nystagmus during the last 10 s in darkness (fig. 1a) and the mean slow-phase velocity of caloric nystagmus in light with eyes fixed for 10 s (fig. 1b) were measured. Visual suppression of caloric nystagmus was calculated as follows:

$$\text{Visual suppression } (\%) = \frac{a-b}{a} \times 100.$$

Results

Visual Suppression in Normal Adults (fig. 1)

Visual suppression of the slow-phase velocity of caloric nystagmus was $66 \pm 11\%$ in 52 normal adults, aged from 21 to 40 years.

Reduced or Abolished Visual Suppression

Visual suppression of caloric nystagmus toward the side of the lesion was reduced or abolished after unilateral flocculus lesions, and

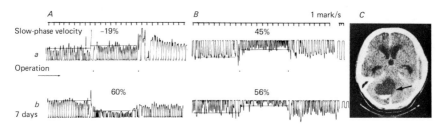

Slow-phase velocity −19%   45%   1 mark/s

a

Operation

b   60%   56%
7 days

Fig. 2. The left cerebellar hemangioblastoma. Visual suppression of caloric nystagmus to the ipsilateral side is abolished and visual suppression of caloric nystagmus to the contralateral side is normal. 7 days after the operation, visual suppression becomes normal bilaterally. *A* Caloric nystagmus to the left. *B* Caloric nystagmus to the right. *C* CT scan (the arrow indicates the lesion). *A, B* and *C* are the same in figures 3–8.

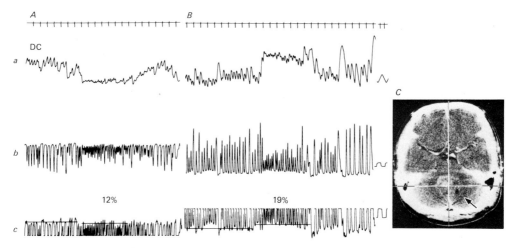

a   DC

b

c   12%   19%

Fig. 3. The astrocytoma of the middle cerebellum. Visual suppression of caloric nystagmus is bilaterally reduced. *a* The eye movement recordings, cal. 10°. *b* The eye speed recordings, cal. 20°/s. *c* The slow-phase velocity, cal. 20°/s. *a, b* and *c* are the same in figures 2–8.

was abolished bilaterally after bilateral flocculus lesions [8]. After nodulus lesions, visual suppression was reduced bilaterally [9].

Visual suppression of caloric nystagmus toward the side of the lesion was abolished and that toward the contralateral side was normal in cases of unilateral cerebellar lesions (fig. 2).

Visual suppression of caloric nystagmus was reduced bilaterally in lesions of the middle part of the cerebellum (fig. 3).

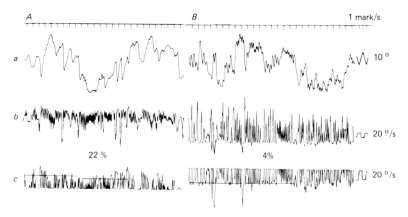

Fig. 4. Spinocerebellar degeneration. Visual suppression of caloric nystagmus is bilaterally reduced.

Visual suppression of caloric nystagmus was reduced or abolished bilaterally in cases of spinocerebellar degeneration (fig. 4), or cerebellitis or diphenylhydantoin intoxication.

Loss of Visual Suppression with
Augmentation of Caloric Nystagmus in Light

When visual suppression was not seen and the caloric nystagmus showed augmentation in light, visual suppression was expressed as –x%. The phenomenon of augmentation of caloric nystagmus in light without visual suppression was seen in cases of pontine lesions or in cases of lower parietal lobe lesions.

In cases of the paramedian pontine reticular formation lesion, the visual suppression of caloric nystagmus to the ipsilateral side vanished and the caloric nystagmus itself became stronger in light than in darkness. However, visual suppression of caloric nystagmus to the contralateral side was normal (fig. 5).

In cases of Millard-Gubler syndrome, visual suppression of caloric nystagmus to the ipsilateral side was abolished and the augmentation of caloric nystagmus in light was seen. Visual suppression of caloric nystagmus to the contralateral side was reduced (fig. 6).

In cases of lower parietal lobe lesions, visual suppression of caloric nystagmus to the ipsilateral side was reduced or abolished and, sometimes, the augmentation of caloric nystagmus in light was seen.

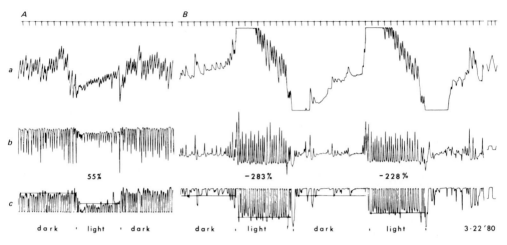

Fig. 5. Pontine glioma with the right paramedian pontine reticular formation (Rt. PPRF) lesion. Visual suppression of caloric nystagmus to the ipsilateral side is abolished and visual suppression of caloric nystagmus to the contralateral side is normal.

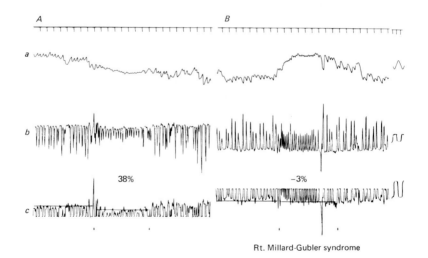

Fig. 6. Right Millard-Gubler syndrome. Visual suppression of caloric nystagmus to the ipsilateral side is abolished and the augmentation of caloric nystagmus is seen in light. Visual suppression of caloric nystagmus to the contralateral side is reduced.

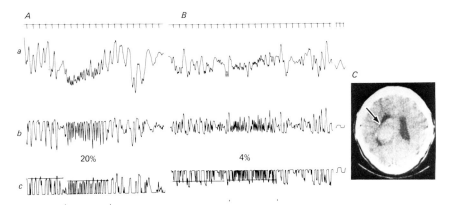

Fig. 7. Left parietal lobe tumor. Visual suppression is bilaterally reduced.

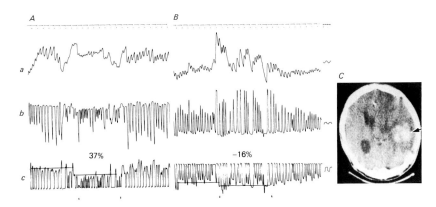

Fig. 8. Right thalamus hemorrhage. Visual suppression of caloric nystagmus to the ipsilateral side is abolished and augmentation of caloric nystagmus is seen in light. Visual suppression of caloric nystagmus to the contralateral side is reduced.

Visual suppression of caloric nystagmus to the contralateral side was sometimes reduced (fig. 7, 8).

In cases of olivopontocerebellar degeneration, visual suppression of caloric nystagmus was abolished and even the augmentation of caloric nystagmus in light was seen.

Visual suppression showed various results, from normal to abolished in cases of idiopathic congenital nystagmus.

Increase of Visual Suppression of Caloric Nystagmus [10]

Visual suppression of caloric nystagmus increased when visual suppression was examined repeatedly in normal subjects, or visual suppressioni gradually increased after unilateral sudden loss of inner ear function. Visual suppression reached 75–80% when the compensation was acquired after unilateral sudden loss of inner ear function.

Discussion

Visual suppression of caloric nystagmus toward the lesion side was reduced after unilateral flocculus lesion and visual suppression of caloric nystagmus to both sides vanished after bilateral flocculus lesions [8]. After nodulus lesions, visual suppression of caloric nystagmus was reduced bilaterally [9]. Visual suppression of caloric nystagmus was reduced or abolished only after flocculus or nodulus lesions in cerebellar lesions, however, visual suppression, seen in cerebellar lesions, never showed augmentation of caloric nystagmus in light [9].

Maekawa and Simpson [5] demonstrated the pathway from the eyes to the flocculus via the inferior olive which was important for the visual suppression mechanism. This may be the main pathway of visual suppression of caloric nystagmus in the cerebellum.

Sometimes, caloric nystagmus was very poor with eyes open in darkness and caloric nystagmus showed the augmentation of its responses in light. This phenomenon was noticed in pontine lesions. The augmentation of caloric nystagmus toward the ipsilateral side was seen in light and visual suppression of caloric nystagmus toward the contralateral side was normal in lesions of the paramedian pontine reticular formation. This augmentation of caloric nystagmus in light was mainly caused by reduced alertness or by disturbance of the quick phase of nystagmus [13].

The absence of visual suppression of caloric nystagmus was also seen in cases of lower parietal lobe lesions [12]. The parietal lobe is very important for visual fixation. Bálint syndrome is known to be caused by lower parietal lobe lesions [1,3].

There seem to be three pathways of concern in the visual fixation mechanism: (1) the eye-flocculus route; (2) the paramedian pontine reticular formation route, and (3) the lower parietal lobe route.

In the lesions of the eye-flocculus route, visual suppression of caloric nystagmus is reduced ipsilaterally. In bilateral lesions, visual suppression is reduced or abolished bilaterally, however, the augmentation of caloric nystagmus in light never appears in lesions of the eye-flocculus route. In cases of paramedian pontine reticular formation lesions, visual suppression is abolished and the augmentation of caloric nystagmus in light is seen. In cases of lower parietal lobe lesions, visual suppression is reduced or abolished and, sometimes, the augmentation of caloric nystagmus is seen.

Conclusion

The phenomenon of visual suppression was found to be influenced by the flocculus or nodulus in the cerebellum [8, 9]. This visual suppression was applied to clinical cases to diagnose the localized lesions in the cerebellum. The following lesions could be diagnosed by this visual suppression test: (1) the flocculus or nodulus lesions in the cerebellum; (2) pontine lesions; (3) lower parietal lobe lesions, and (4) compensation after unilateral sudden loss of inner ear function.

References

1   Bálint, R.: Seelenlähmung des «Schauens», optische Ataxie, räumliche Störung der Aufmerksamkeit. Mschr. Psychiat. Neurol. 25: 51–81 (1909).
2   Frenzel, H.: Spontan- und Provokations-Nystagmus als Krankheitssymptom (Springer, Berlin, 1955).
3   Hécaen, H.; Ajuriaguerra, J. de: Balint syndrome (psychic paralysis of visual fixation) and its minor forms. Brain 77: 373–400 (1974).
4   Mahoney, J.L.; Harlan, W.L.; Bickford, R.G.: Visual and other factors influencing caloric nystagmus in normal subjects. Archs Otolar. 66: 46–53 (1957).
5   Maekawa, K.; Simpson, J.L.: Climbing fiber responses evoked in vestibulo-cerebellum of rabbit from visual system. J. Neurophysiol. 86: 649–666 (1973).
6   Ohm, J.: Über den Einfluss des Sehens auf den vestibulären Drehnystagmus und Nachnystagmus. Z. Hals-Nasen-Ohrenheilk. 16: 521–540 (1926).
7   Takemori S.; Cohen, B.: Visual suppression of vestibular nystagmus in rhesus monkeys. Brain Res. 72: 203–212 (1974).
8   Takemori, S.; Cohen, B.: Loss of visual suppression of vestibular nystagmus after flocculus lesions. Brain Res. 72: 213–224 (1974).
9   Takemori, S.: Visual suppression of vestibular nystagmus after cerebellar lesions. Annls Oto-lar. 84: 318–326 (1975).

10 Takemori, S.: Increase of visual suppression of vestibular nystagmus in rhesus monkeys; in Morimoto, Proc. 5th Extraordinary Meet. Bárány Soc., pp. 91–95 (Japan Society for Equilibrium Research, Tokyo 1975).
11 Takemori, S.: Visual suppression test. Clin. Otolaryngol. *3:* 145–153 (1978).
12 Takemori, S.; Ono, M.; Maeda, T.: Cerebral contribution to the visual suppression of vestibular nystagmus. Archs Otolar. *105:* 579–581 (1979).
13 Takemori, S.; Aiba, T.; Shiozawa, R.: Visual-vestibular interaction: visual suppression of caloric nystagmus in brain stem lesions. Ann. N.Y. Acad. Sci. *374:* 846–854 (1981).

Dr. S. Takemori, Neurotology, Toranomon Hospital, Toranomon 2-2-2, Minato-Ku, Tokyo 107 (Japan)

Adv. Oto-Rhino-Laryng., vol. 29, pp. 111–123 (Karger, Basel 1983)

Vestibular Neuronitis –
Its Clinical Characteristics

Toru Sekitani

Department of Otolaryngology, Yamaguchi University, School of Medicine,
Ube City, Japan

An attack of vertigo in the vestibular neuronitis is seemingly similar to vertiginous attacks of Ménière's disease, with several differences in the clinical features between them [1–3]. The clinical picture of vestibular neuronitis is characterized by strong and single attacks of vertigo with some vestibular impairment but without any cochlear impairment [4–6]; unsteadiness of gait continued in the majority of patients and 'disturbed sensation of body balance' remains for a period of time [9] from several months to years). In some cases, the onset of dizziness was preceded by mild to moderate increases in temperature, ill feeling with general fatigue, and evidence of upper respiratory infection. Also, there are other clinical features in neurotology, including canal paresis by the caloric test and peculiar patterns (response) in computed galvanic body-sway tests; the latter suggesting a retrolabyrinthine disorder.

The purpose of this paper is mainly to discuss the results of an epidemiological survey on vestibular neuronitis in Japan, based on the findings of a preliminary survey and a programmed nationwide survey. Secondly this paper will present the results of a galvanic body-sway test for differential diagnosis of this disease's entity and to evaluate the progress and prognosis of this disease.

Diagnostic Criteria

Before reporting on the data presented in this paper, clinical diagnostic criteria must be determined to define the disease. To comple-

Table I. Characteristic clinical features of vestibular Neuronitis[1]

---

1 Vertigo, but not always paroxysmal in character:
  1–2: sudden and transient seizures with sensation of 'blackout'
  1–3 'feeling top-heavy' or 'off-balance', particularly when walking or standing
2 Conspicuous absence of cochlear signs
3 Suspected lesion: some form of organic disease; in the peripheral nervous pathways,
  up to the vestibular nuclei in the brainstem
4 Age: chiefly affects the 30–50 age group
5 Sex: no preference
6 Some kind of febrile illness, or with evidence of infection of the ears, nose and throat
7 Marked abnormalities, always present: *reduced caloric response*
  (complete – severe – moderate canal paresis)
8 No evidence of extravestibular nervous disease
9 *Galvanic test response* (reduced); indicative of a lesion central to Scarpa's ganglion
10 Essentially benign; it responds well to treatment of focal infection
  (when this is present)

---

[1] This tabulation is made from *Dix and Hallpike's* original description [cf.16].

Table II. Diagnostic criteria as 'important clinical facts' in vestibular neuronitis (after *Stahle* [7])

---

1 Younger people
2 Following an infection
3 Acute onset of dizziness
4 Protracted course
5 Benign lesion in the peripheral pathways
6 Unilateral in most case
7 Reduced caloric excitability
8 Spontaneous nystagmus beating away from diseased labyrinth
9 Reduced galvanic response
10 Normal hearing; no tinnitus
11 Normal CSF; normal EEG
12 Therapy symptomatic

---

ment the original descriptions of the 100 cases of vestibular neuronitis by *Dix and Hallpike* [4], there are many other outstanding descriptions regarding the criteria of this disease. But, due to various interpretations of the clinical features on vestibular neuronitis and excessive transcriptions of the original papers, some confusion in the so-called criteria arose. There was no definite dividing line between the original descrip-

Table III. Diagnostic criteria of vestibular neuronitis (by Vestibular Disorders Research Committee, Japan, 1980)

---

1 Vertiginous attack (as chief complaint); single attack in most cases
2 Hypo- or null-reaction to caloric stimulation of labyrinth
   (unilateral–bilateral)
3 No abnormality of cochlear and central nervous system

Additional comment
1 Proceeding 'upper respiratory infection' and sign of common colds
2 None of disease related to the vertigo
3 Reduced or null response to galvanic test

---

tion of the clinical feature and any additional comments by either researchers.

I would like to mention several descriptions relating the clinical criteria. The original description of vestibular neuronitis by *Dix and Hallpike* [4] were tabulated and shown in table I, which closely follows the original description (table I). Secondly, *Stahle*'s [7] 'important clinical facts of the vestibular neuritis' is also of importance with each heading and in the same order as shown in table II. Thirdly, there is the diagnostic criteria reported by the Research Team on Peripheral Vestibular Disorders sponsored by the Ministry of Health and Welfare in Japan; applying the systematic nationwide survey on peripheral vestibular disorders (including vestibular neuronitis) (table III).

Epidemiological Survey (Preliminary Survey;
Collected at Yamaguchi University Hospital)

A preliminary report of an epidemiological survey of vestibular neuronitis was made using a simple questionnaire [11]. Postcards were distributed to 56 medical facilities throughout Japan, responses were gathered from 33 facilities (58.9%) (including otoneurological clinics of university hospitals and outstanding district hospitals) (fig. 1). During the 3-year period from January 1975 to December 1977, 25,512 patients were examined otoneurologically at these 33 medical facilities. Of those examined, 412 were diagnosed as having vestibular neuronitis (1.6% on average: 1.2% in 1975, 1.5% in 1976, and 2.1% in 1977). These

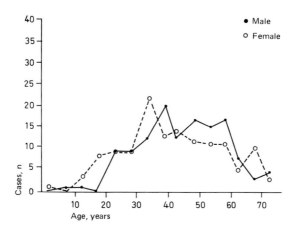

Fig. 1. Vestibular neuronitis – occurrence in age and sex of 412 cases collected from 33 medical facilities in Japan (1975–1977) by the questionnaire method. Note: the youngest were a 5-year-old girl and 7-year-old boy; the oldest was a 77-year-old male.

Table IV. Nationwide survey on 'vestibular neuronitis'

	Patients with vertigo, examined	VN	%
1975	7,789	92	1.2
1976	8,426	125	1.5
1977	9,301	195	2.1
	25,516	412	1.6

Questionnaire to 56 major hospitals (including University Hospital and Regional Medical Centers); answers from 33 facilities (58.9%).

patients consisted of 220 males and 192 females, a distribution of 53.4 and 46.6%, respectively. The affected side was, right 207 (50.2%), left 180 (43.7%), and bilateral 25 (6.1%). A preliminary survey of seasonal occurrence suggested periodicity in the occurrence of the disease every 4 months, although this has not yet been completely clarified. A further epidemiological survey of vestibular neuronitis is greatly needed under a well-designed and sufficiently controlled scheme involving facilities throughout Japan.

So, a systematic nationwide survey on 'peripheral vestibular disorders' (including vestibular neuronitis) was done in 1980 as one of the

Table V. Nationwide survey of cases with 'vestibular function disorders' (peripheral type)

	Cases
Ménière's disease (definite; incl. 7 susp.)	606
Sudden deafness	227
Vestibular neuronitis	*189*
Benign paroxys. posit vertigo	379
Bilat. vestibul. dysfunction	59
Syphilis, labyrinth	22
Traumatic vestib. involvement	68
	1,550

Occurence rate of the vestibular neuronitis in so-called 'peripheral vestibular disorders'. Cases are collected as systematic nationwide survey in 1980 of Japan by Research Committee (cf.12).

series of research projects of the Vestibular Disorder Research Committee, Ministry of Health and Welfare, Japan (the author acts as one of the members). In the 1981 annual report, *Watanabe*[12] reported the incidence of each peripheral vestibular disorder (table III). According to this report, vestibular neuronitis occurred in 189 (12.2%) of 1,550 patients registered in the survey. We must pay attention to the numbers – 189 patients who were diagnosed as having vestibular neuronitis compared to 606 with Ménière disease (which is an unexpectedly higher occurrence compared with other previous reports) (table IV, V).

Galvanic Body-Sway Test (Method and Results) [10, 13]

Head- and body-sway elicited by galvanic stimulation on the mastoid area was recorded by two small accelerometers on a helmet worn by the subjects. Weak galvanic stimulation was usually 0.6 mA, induced by a unilateral anodal electrode on the right and/or left mastoid area. The bilateral-unipolar method was used later. A computer was used to average the responses to 8–16 repeated stimuli. The analysis time for each response was 10–20 s. The current stimulus started at the point of 1 s after the analysis began and lasted for 5–10 s (see the legend of figure 2). Figures 2 and 3 show the actual record of the computed galvanic body-sway test of a subject with vestibular neuronitis. Inter-

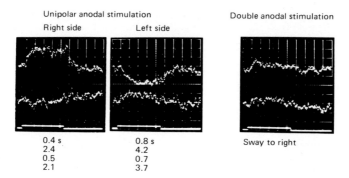

Unipolar anodal stimulation

Right side   Left side

Double anodal stimulation

Sway to right

0.4 s	0.8 s
2.4	4.2
0.5	0.7
2.1	3.7

Fig. 2. Computed galvanic body-sway test (Yamaguchi University). Representative record of a 18-year-old woman with left-sided vestibular neuronitis. Anodal stimulation (0.6 mA for 10 s) through the electrode on the left retroauricular skin induced 'slow body deviation' to the left (in the middle of the figure). Note: movement of the head and body toward the right side is expressed as upward deflection of the trace in the acceleration-registrography. Interval B, for example, 2.4 ms on right side, is a time length of the induced head-body deviation. On the contrary, interval B of the left side is 4.2 ms i.e., 'slow and sluggish response'.

vals A, B, C and D were all markedly prolonged with left-sided anodal stimulation. This pattern indicates that the progress of the body-sway is relatively slower after galvanic stimulation than that of the opposite, healthy side. This 'delayed' response to stimulation on the affected side is frequently seen in vestibular neuronitis, with some peculiarity in the disease, but less frequently seen in other vertiginous diseases. This fact indicates some unique feature of pathognomosis of this disease entity. With bilateral anodal stimulation, the record showed body-sway to the right, the healthy side due to hyporeactivity on the left side (the far right side of figure 2).

Evaluation of Prognosis

Clinical examinations, including the galvanic body-sway tests, were performed twice in each of 10 patients with vestibular neuronitis during the course of the illness. Observation periods varied from 1 month to 6 years, averaging 24.7 months. In figure 4, data for one case of a computed galvanic body-sway test is shown. In this figure, time length of section B was dominantly prolonged in the affected side compared with the healthy side at the time of 'shortly after onset'. This prolongation is yielded by a slow, sluggish response of body deviation

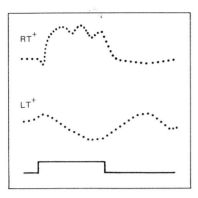

Fig. 3. Graphic presentation of the records of computed galvanic body-sway test. The lowest line: mark of galvanic stimulation. The uppermost record: (RT+) means 'anodal stimulation on the right side (healthy ear in this case). The dotted line of the uppermost showed the computer-averaged curve of the body-sway to the right side, induced by galvanic stimulation. The middle record: (LT+) anodal stimulation on the left ear (affected side). Note the definite 'slow response of the induced body deviation'.

induced by galvanic stimulation. This abnormally slow response no longer existed at the 5-year check. Figure 4 also shows no notable change in the results of the healthy-side stimulation. Therefore, the galvanic test will evaluate the disease's process and prognosis.

In figure 5, a summary of the follow-up results in interval B of computed galvanic body-sway tests is shown, obtained from 10 cases with vestibular neuronitis. For example, (1) improvement of the abnormal pattern was observed in 7 patients, (2) no marked change was observed in 1 case, and (3) a prolonged interval B was present in 2 cases. 2 of these 10 patients still experience a slight sensation of instability.

Case 1

The patient was a 37-year-old female, who first visited our clinic on March 31, 1979. Her chief complaints were attacks of rotatory vertigo and nausea. 2 days prior to admission she felt a sudden attack of rotatory vertigo. This attack had been preceded by rhinorrhea and nasal obstruction for 1 week. No vomiting or severe headache was reported.

Vestibular function tests were performed on the first day of visit (fig. 6). Mann's test and the goniometer test could not be performed due to the patient's difficulty in standing. In the vertical writing test

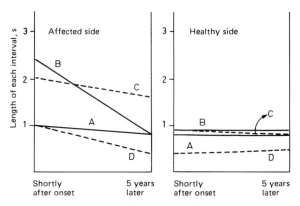

Fig. 4. Prognosis of vestibular neuronitis. Data of computed galvanic body-sway test in both period of 'shortly after onset' and of '5 years after'; comparing every section of the record which was obtained in case of anodal stimulation in each ear (healthy and affected side).

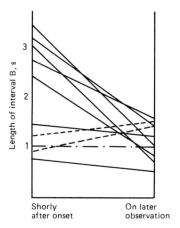

Fig. 5. Follow-up results on interval B of the record of computed galvanic body-sway test. 10 cases with vestibular neuronitis showed prolonged interval B when tested shortly after the onset. In the data of the follow-up examination, there are 7 cases which showed 'recovering to the normal range'; 1 unchanged and 2 cases showed 'slightly prolonged to worse'.

(copying her name in Chinese characters in a vertical column), the line of written letters deviated to the left side and was detected with the micrographism. OKP and ETT were within normal limits. Spontaneous nystagmus, recorded by ENG, was horizontal and direction-fixed to the right side even when opposite the direction of the gaze. Spontane-

Date: Jan. 19, 1978
Case: 37-year-old female
Diagnosis: vestibular neuronitis on the left side

Romberg: within normal limit
Mann: falling with eyes closed
Writing: micrographism and shortening
ETT: irregular pattern slightly
OKP: central suppression slightly

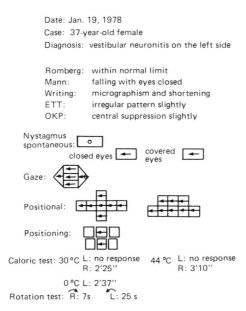

Caloric test: 30 °C L: no response   44 °C L: no response
              R: 2'25"   R: 3'10"

              0 °C L: 2'37"
Rotation test: R: 7s   L: 25 s

Fig. 6. Otoneurological findings in case of vestibular neuronitis.

ous nystagmus was observed in both positional and positioning tests. Caloric tests revealed canal paresis on the left side. Audiometry showed no present reduction of hearing acuity, nor did it show a reduction during any of the three follow-up examinations; 2–4 days after onset, 2 months and 6 months later. No other neurological signs suggesting central lesion were noted.

Discussion

Vestibular neuronitis is a problematic disease entity. There are several different names in terminology. Definite terminology is necessary to understand the disease itself. And there are also quite a number of questions about the disease: What is its cause? What is the pathognomosis, and is it completely understood and acceptable? How is the epidemiology in a problem? What are the pathophysiological changes within the vestibular system? Which are the best, and/or advisable tests for diagnosis? And how should we treat a patient with vestibular

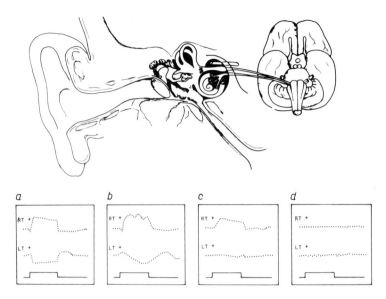

Fig. 7. Representative diagram of the results of computed galvanic body-sway test. For topographical diagnosis in the vestibular nervous system, the findings consist of: *(a)* otitis media chronica, without any detectable abnormality in the inner ear (similar to the healthy subject); *(b)* vestibular neuronitis; *(c)* acoustic neuroma; *(d)* congenital deaf-mute (no response to sound and to the ice water caloric stimulation).

neuronitis? All of these problems are not completely solved yet at the clinical level.

We would emphasize the recognition of the name of this disease itself and of the diagnostic criteria originating from the description by *Dix and Hallpike* [4]. Definite diagnosis of vestibular neuronitis among the so-called vertiginous patients is also necessary. As pointed out by *Dix and Hallpike* [4] in 1952, the use of galvanic tests in vestibular neuronitis is highly effective for differentiating between these retrolabyrinthine disorders from the vertigo, the causes of which lie in the vestibular system, and for evaluating the prognosis of the disease. We have also recognized the usefulness of this test and have studied various kinds of galvanic tests in clinics and laboratories for more than 20 years [10]. Recently, we have used this method in clinics as a routine test in forms of computed galvanic body-sway test [10].

In figure 7, a representative diagram of the results of computed galvanic body-sway test (Yamaguchi University) was illustrated for to-

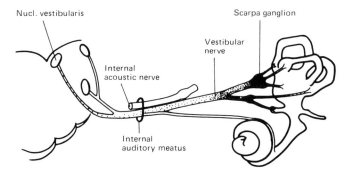

Fig. 8. Histopathological finding in the vestibular neuronitis [after *Morgenstein and Seung,* 8].

pographical diagnosis in the vestibular nervous system. The findings in these figures consist of: (1) otitis media chronica with a purely conductive type hearing loss but without any detectable abnormality in the inner ear (the findings are similar to those of healthy subjects); (2) vestibular neuronitis, showing a peculiar slow response of deviation of his head and body, (3) acoustic neuroma, and (4) congenital deaf-mute with dead labyrinths. As indicated in figure 7, the case of vestibular neuronitis showed a peculiar response in the body-sway induced by weak galvanic stimulation, suggesting unusual characteristics and a different reaction level of the nerve fibers in the vestibulospinal system.

According to *Morgenstein and Seung* [8], the histopathological findings in the vestibular nervous system in cases with vestibular neuronitis are mainly scattered degenerative changes in the Scarpa's ganglion, vestibular nerve and in the central nerve, close to the vestibular nucleus. These changes are presented in figure 8.

Recently, *Schuknecht and Kitamura* [3] described in detail and discussed vestibular neuritis. Their description was as follows: histopathological evidence in the temporal bones of 4 subjects supports the existence of a discrete degenerative neuropathy of the vestibular nerve. The pathological correlates as determined by temporal bone studies is the result of atrophy of one or more vestibular nerve trunks, with or without their associated sense organs. *Schuknecht and Kitamura* [3] also suspected that viral etiology was the cause of the disease. Speaking of viral etiology, we also have an interesting case with an attack of vertigo which takes a similar course of vestibular neuronitis after influenza vaccination [15].

Morinaka and Yoshinobu [14] also reported a case of vestibular neuronitis with periodical changes in the serum titer of herpes simplex. Little information has as yet been gathered and reported. These discrete degenerative changes in the nerve fibers in the vestibular nerve trunks yield a scattered and delayed impulse conduction along the vestibular nerves and produces slow responses of the nerve's excitability to the galvanic stimulation.

Further clinical systematic studies of this disease are necessary in clinical and in histopathological laboratories to advance seroimmunology.

Summary

Several parts of a nationwide survey of the epidemiology of vestibular neuronitis were reported. Follow-up studies of vestibular neuronitis were made. The computed galvanic body-sway test (Yamaguchi University) obtained from 10 patients with vestibular neuronitis showed a peculiar 'slow and sluggish' pattern. In the course of the illness, this slow and sluggish pattern changed its appearance and soon resembled the pattern obtained from the opposite, healthy side. Improvement of the abnormal pattern was observed in 7 patients (observation period 6 months to 6 years, averaging 33 months). 3 other patients (observation period 1 month to 1 year, averaging 5.3 months) showed no improvement in the pattern.

These findings suggest that the conductivity of the vestibular nerve affected by vestibular neuronitis has an increasing chance for recovery.

References

1 Ruttin, B.: Zur Differentialdiagnose der Labyrinth und Hörnerverkrankungen. Z. Ohrenheilk. *57:* 327–331 (1909).
2 Nylen, C.: Some cases of ocular nystagmus due to certain positions of the head. Acta oto-lar. *6:* 106–123 (1924).
3 Schuknecht, H.F.; Kitamura, K.: Vestibular neuritis. Ann. Otol. Rhinol. *90:* suppl. 78, pp 1–19 (1981).
4 Dix, M.R.; Hallpike, C.S.: The pathology, symptomatology and diagnosis of certain common disorders of the vestibular system. Ann. Otol. Rhinol. Lar. *61:* 987–1017 (1952).
5 Pfaltz, C.R.: Diagnose und Therapie der vestibulären Neuronitis. Pract. oto-rhinolar. *17:* 454–461 (1955).
6 Watanabe, I.: Ménière's syndrome without cochlear symptom (in Japanese). ORL, Tokyo *2:* 234 (1959).

7 Stahle, J.: Vestibular neuritis; in Wolfson, The vestibular system and its disease (University of Pennsylvania Press, Philadelphia 1966).

8 Morgenstein, K.M.; Seung, I.S.: Vestibular neuronitis. Laryngoscope *81:* 131–139 (1971).

9 Sekitani, T.: Vestibular neuritis. Bull. Yamaguchi med. School *22:* 317–324 (1975).

10 Sekitani, T.; Tanaka, M.: Test for galvanic vestibular response – Survey through our experimental and clinical investigations for the last 20 years. Bull. Yamaguchi Med. School *22:* 439–452 (1975).

11 Sekitani, T., et al.: An epidemiological study of vestibular neuronitis – a preliminary report (in Japanese). Pract. Otol., Kyoto *75:* suppl. 1, pp. 193–198 (1982): Annual Report of the Vestibular Disorder Research Committee, Ministry of Health and Welfare, Japan 1980.

12 Watanabe, I.: First report of the nationwide epidemiological survey on the vestibular disorder in Japan (in Japanese). Annual Report of the Vestibular Disorder Research Committee, Ministry of Health and Welfare, Japan 1980, pp. 39–46.

13 Okuzono, T.; Sekitani,T., et al.: Computed galvanic body sway test – peculiarity in vestibular neuronitis. Postural reflex and body equilibrium No. 2, pp. 97–105 (Society of Nara Neurotological Research, Nara 1981).

14 Morinaka, S.; Yoshinobu, T.: A vertiginous patient with vestibular neuritis related to herpes simplex infection – with reference to the results of equilibrium test and virological-serological examinations (in Japanese). Pract. Otol., Kyoto *74:* 1523–1535 (1981).

15 Hiyoshi, M.; Sekitani, T., et al.: Vertigo consistent with the so-called vestibular neuronitis after influenza vaccination (in Japanese). Pract. Otol., Kyoto *75:* suppl. 1, pp. 260–265 (1982).

16 Sekitani, T.: List of literature on vestibular neuronitis. Pract. Otol., Kyoto (in press, 1982).

Prof. T. Sekitani, MD, Department of Otolaryngology, Yamaguchi University, School of Medicine, Ube City 755 (Japan)

Adv. Oto-Rhino-Laryng., vol. 29, pp. 124–139 (Karger, Basel 1983)

Electric Response Audiometry: The Morphology of Normal Responses

Jon K. Shallop

Department of Otolaryngology and Head and Neck Surgery, Indiana University School of Medicine, Indianapolis, Ind., USA

The idea of evoking electrical potentials in response to sound from the human auditory pathways has been with us now for at least 50 years. However, the improved technology of recent years has made it more feasible to accurately record the various auditory evoked potentials and to make them clinically applicable for audiometric purposes *Davis*, 1976; *Picton* et al., 1977]. The term electric response audiometry (ERA) has been adopted by the International Electric Response Audiometry Study Group and it will be utilized in this paper. ERA encompasses all of the various electrical potentials which can be measured from the human auditory pathways in response to sound stimuli. These responses are then used to predict the audiometric status of a particular child or adult. Some of the auditory evoked potentials, especially the brainstem responses, are of major interest to neurologists in the diagnosis of various neurological problems. However, this paper will be limited to audiometric applications of auditory evoked potentials.

Historically, ERA has developed from the two anatomical extremes of the auditory system. The first measured auditory potentials were the cortically evoked potentials, which ultimately became clinically more useful with the development of the signal averagers which became commercially available in the 1960s. An example of the auditory cortical evoked response is illustrated in figure 1. The reader is cautioned to note the various notations for all figures in this paper. Specifically note whether the voltages are expressed as positive or negative upward, note the time scale of the particular response and also note the

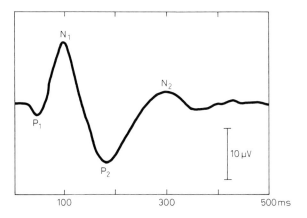

Fig. 1. The slow vertex (cortical) auditory evoked potential typically has at least four prominent peaks as indicated. Note that negative polarity is referenced upward and that the time window is 500 ms [*Fria* et al., 1979].

relative amplitude of the response voltage which is usually indicated with a calibration voltage.

The cortical auditory potential illustrated in figure 1 has four prominent peaks labelled: P_1, N_1, P_2 and N_2. The N_1-P_2 waves have been typically used as the main feature indicating auditory threshold. The slow vertex (cortical) response to decreasing sound levels is illustrated in figure 2 [*Fria* et al., 1979]. Figure 2 demonstrates a general principle that will be noted throughout this paper in that the response amplitudes decrease and the response latencies increase, as the sound stimuli are attenuated (dB HL). Note that in figure 2 a response to the 1,000 Hz toneburst can be observed down to 5–10 dB HL.

The late cortical evoked auditory potentials have not become standard clinical tools for hearing assessment because they are affected dramatically by sleep state, as illustrated in figure 3 [*Osterhammel* et al., 1973]. Note that in the deeper stages of sleep, the responses become more variable.

The next auditory evoked potential to be discussed will be the middle latency responses (MLR) which were first described as the fast vertex responses. A sample MLR is presented in figure 4 [*Brown and Shallop*,1981]. The most prominent feature of the MLR is generally the P_a wave which has a latency of 30–35 ms at moderate sensation levels. Figure 4 also shows an MLR intensity series for a 500 Hz toneburst. The P_a

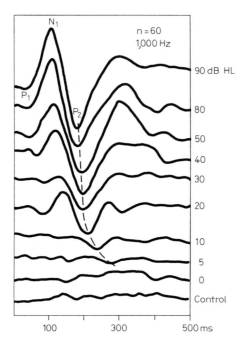

Fig. 2. The slow vertex response from an adult with normal hearing illustrates the changes in response morphology as the sound level is attenuated toward threshold. In this instance we would predict that hearing is normal at 1,000 Hz for the ear tested [*Fria* et al., 1979].

peak can be observed down to 25 dB HL and perhaps there is a response at 15 dB HL for this particular patient. The middle components are also affected by sleep state as illustrated in figure 5 [*Brown and Shallop,* 1981]. Note the decreased amplitudes and the waveform morphology changes of the MLR in the various sleep states.

Recently, *Galambos* et al. [1981] have described a procedure for enhancing the middle component responses. This technique requires the sequential presentation of tonebursts or clicks at a rate of 40/s in order to optimize the response [fig. 6]. Note that each toneburst evokes an MLR and if these responses are then summed with the signal averager,

Fig. 4. The middle latency response (MLR) is shown for an adult with normal hearing at 500 Hz. The various positive polarity waves of the response are indicated. Note that a response can be detected at 15 dB [*Brown and Shallop,* 1981].

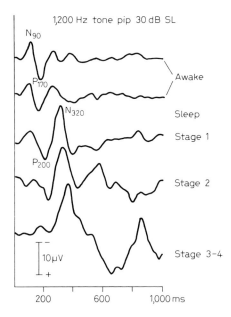

1,200 Hz tone pip 30 dB SL

N90

P170

N320

P200

10 μV

Awake

Sleep

Stage 1

Stage 2

Stage 3-4

200   600   1,000 ms

Fig. 3. The slow vertex response morphology is altered dramatically as a result of the sleep state of the person tested. This fact makes this auditory evoked potential unreliable when subjects are in natural or sedated sleep [*Osterhammel* et al., 1973].

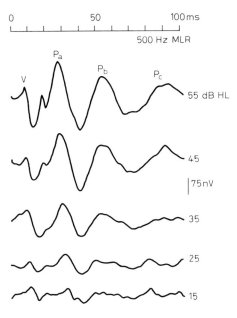

0   50   100 ms

500 Hz MLR

Pa

V   Pb   Pc

55 dB HL

45

75 nV

35

25

15

Fig. 4

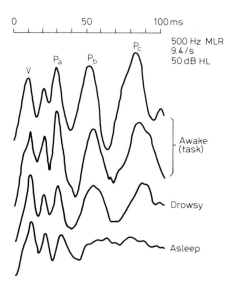

Fig. 5. The middle latency response (MLR) is shown for an adult with normal hearing at 500 Hz in various stages of attention/sleep. The 500 Hz toneburst (4-2-4 ms) was presented at 50 dB HL. There is an obvious change in the morphology of the response which causes a reduction in the amplitudes, especially P_a and P_b [*Brown and Shallop, 1981*].

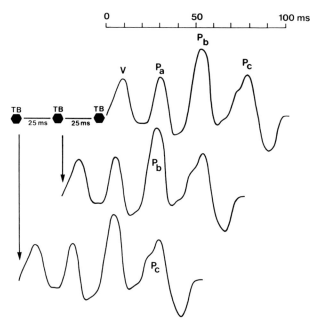

Fig. 6

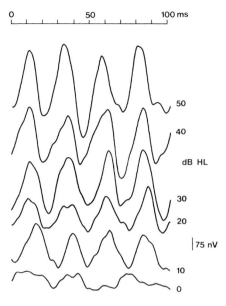

0 ├─┴─┴─┴─┴─┤ 50 ├─┴─┴─┴─┴─┤ 100 ms

50

40

dB HL

30

20

│75 nV

10

0

Fig. 7. The 40/s MLR resultant waveform from an adult with normal hearing demonstrates the large amplitudes obtained with this technique. Note the apparent response at 10 dB HL.

a response as illustrated in figure 7 is obtained. This response may also be useful in the prediction of hearing sensitivity since it can be observed at low sensation levels. [*Brown and Shallop*, 1981]. Figure 8 demonstrates the 40/s MLR from an adult with a low- to mid-frequency sensorineural hearing loss. Note that the 40/s MLR predicted threshold would be 40–50 dB HL, which is in excellent agreement with the actual audiogram from this patient obtained on the same day. The auditory brainstem response (ABR) to unfiltered clicks is illustrated in the upper left of figure 8. This response will be described later in this paper.

Figure 9 illustrates another adult with a low-frequency sensorineural hearing loss. Again note the good agreement between the 40/s MLR

Fig. 6. The paradigm for the 40/s MLR is shown as it has been described by *Galambos* et al. [1981]. Sequential tonebursts (TB) will evoke overlapping middle latency responses and the summed responses will appear as shown in figure 7.

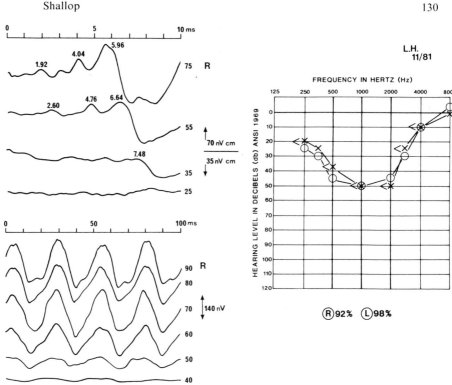

Fig. 8. The ABR and 40/s MLR results are shown for a young woman who has a bilateral mid-frequency sensorineural hearing loss. The ABR for an unfiltered click and the 40/s MLR for a 500 Hz toneburst (4-2-4 ms) are in good agreement with the behavioral audiogram.

and the actual audiometric threshold at 500 Hz. An example of a high-frequency sensorineural hearing loss is presented in figure 10. The results shown in figures 8–10 demonstrate that this particular response is probably a good index of low-frequency hearing. A comparison between the standard MLR and the 40/s MLR is presented in figure 11 [*Brown and Shallop*, 1981]. The main differences noted between these responses are the larger amplitudes of the 40/s responses due to the summing effect of the 40/s MLR.

Fig. 10. The ABR and 40/s MLR results are displayed for an adult with a high-frequency sensorineural hearing loss. Note that the ABR occurs only at 85–95 dB HL. The 40/s MLR accurately predicts the behavioral threshold at 500 Hz.

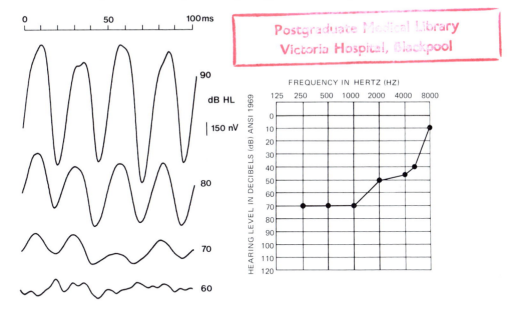

Fig. 9. The 40/s MLR results for a 500 Hz toneburst agree well with the behavioral threshold at 500 Hz.

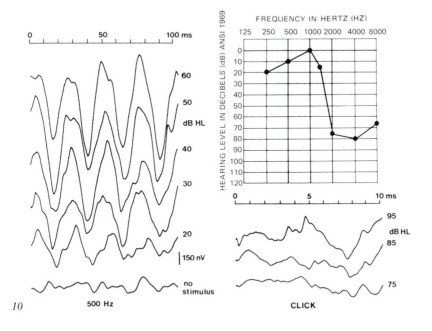

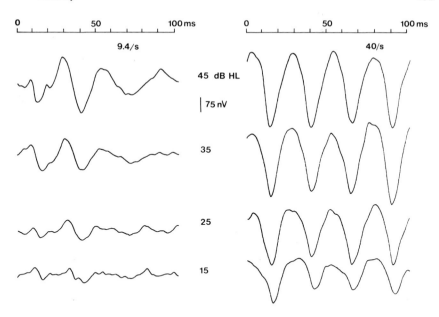

Fig. 11. The standard MLR and the 40/s MLR are compared for the same adult with normal hearing. Note the amplitude differences in the responses [*Brown and Shallop*, 1981].

The auditory brainstem response (ABR/BSER) has probably received the most attention in the past few years of all of the auditory evoked potentials. This response is illustrated in figure 12 [*Fria*, 1980] with vertex positive being upward. The Roman numerals (I–VII) refer to the most prominent features ['waves'] of this response in humans as it was described by *Jewett and Williston* [1971]. Other authors had also described this response earlier in the 1960s [*Sohmer and Feinmesser*, 1967; *Yoshie*, 1968]. The prominent negative potential following wave V in figure 12 is designated FFP-7 and it was described by *Terkildsen* et al. [1973] as another prominent feature of the ABR.

In figure 12 the time scale is 10 ms and this figure also illustrates the peripheral conduction time from stimulus onset to wave I of the ABR, which probably represents activity in the auditory nerve. Central conduction time in the auditory neural tracts of the brainstem is indicated as the response time interval between the auditory nerve (wave I) and about the level of the inferior colliculus (wave V). At a moderate

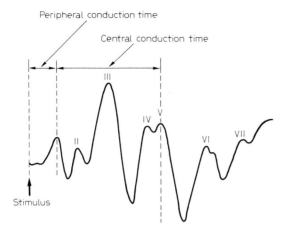

Fig. 12. The auditory brainstem response (ABR) is illustrated. The various waves are indicated with Roman numerals I–VII. This is the typical waveform morphology that would be expected for a moderate level stimulus (60 dB HL) in an adult with normal hearing [*Fria* et al., 1979].

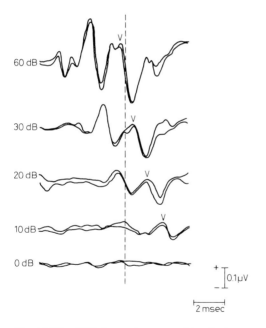

Fig. 13. The ABR for various sound levels demonstrates the changes in waveform morphology which occur as the sound level is decreased. Note the latency shift of wave V [*Fria* et al., 1979].

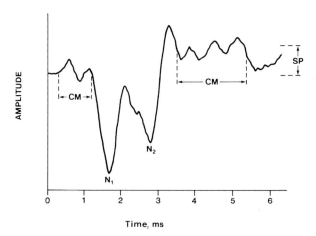

Fig. 16. The averaged whole nerve action potential is shown resulting from ECoG with a round-window electrode in a chinchilla. There are two large negative potentials (N_1 and N_2) observed. The cochlear microphonic (CM) and summating potential (SP) are also apparent in this response.

sponses obtained from 'normal' newborns and infants. Whenever an infant is neurologically abnormal, waveform latencies and morphology must be interpreted carefully.

An example of a normal newborn ABR is illustrated in figure 15. Note that the time scale is 20 ms. A prominent feature of this response is what *Davis and Hirsh* [1979] called the slow negative wave at 10 ms (SN–10). They feel that this wave can be used to aid in the estimation of audiometric thresholds. The recording of this response requires the extension of the high-pass setting on the EEG preamplifier down to about 30 Hz. Typically for most ABR recordings this filter setting is higher, in the range of 100–300 Hz.

The frequency-following response (FFR) was described by *Worden and Marsh* [1968] and it has been considered by various investigators as a possible response that would enable the recording of an evoked potential for low-frequency sounds, i.e. below 1,000 Hz. There appear to be two major problems with this potential: it can only be recorded at levels above 30–40 dB HL and this potential is probably generated in the basal turn of the cochlea. To date this potential has not been widely accepted as a clinically useful measurement of low-frequency hearing.

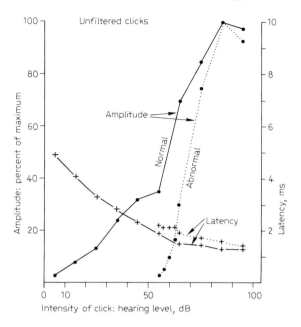

Fig. 17. The ECoG results are shown for a normal hearing person and a person with a 50–60 dB HL sensorineural hearing loss. Latency values are referenced to the left ordinate and the normalized amplitudes are referenced to the right ordinate. The stimulus was an unfiltered click [*Aran*, 1971].

The last potentials to be discussed result from electrical activity in the auditory nerve and the cochlea. The whole nerve action potentials of the auditory nerve can be measured with the same so-called 'far-field' electrodes which are used to obtain all of the evoked potentials described so far in this paper. However, this potential can be recorded with much larger amplitudes by placing one of the active electrodes in the ear canal or on the promontory of the middle ear. The latter procedure is invasive and painful to the patient and it is not used universally as a clinical tool. This 'near-field' placement of an active electrode through the tympanic membrane is called electrocochleography (ECoG). An example of a recorded ECoG response from the round window of a chinchilla is shown in figure 16. The tracing demonstrates the whole nerve action potentials N_1 and N_2 which probably are components of the first wave of the ABR. Figure 16 also illustrates the cochlear microphonic and summating potentials of the cochlea. These

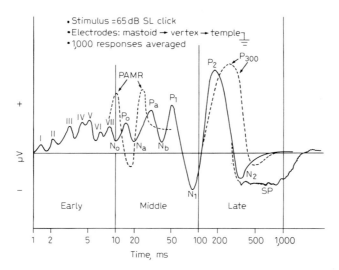

Fig. 18. The various auditory evoked potentials are summarized and displayed in their temporal sequence on a log scale [adapted from *Picton* et al., 1977].

potentials will not be described in any detail, but the reader is referred to *Davis* [1976] for additional information and references.

When human ECoG responses are measured and plotted, they usually are shown as illustrated in figure 17 [*Aran*, 1971]. The maximum amplitude of the action potentials N_1 is normalized to 100% and all other responses are plotted in reference as a percentage of the maximum voltage (in this case 90 dB HL). Additionally, the latencies of the action potential responses are shown and the reader will note that there is a latency range of about 3.0 ms for the normal subject (1.7 ms at 90–95 dB and 4.7 ms at 5–10 dB). This is the same latency range which we observe in the human ABR. An example of a person with a sensorineural hearing loss is also shown in figure 17.

Auditory evoked potentials are known to be of considerable value in the clinical estimation of hearing loss. This paper has reviewed most of the auditory evoked potentials which are summarized and illustrated in figure 18, which is adapted from *Picton* et al. [1977]. This representation of auditory evoked potentials may help the reader conceptualize the various auditory evoked potentials. Note that time is represented on a log scale and the amplitudes are arbitrary, but relative when comparing the various responses.

Acknowledgements

The author expresses his thanks to colleagues and staff in the ENT department for their help in the preparation of this paper, especially *C. Faux, D. Brown, K. Young* and *R. Chaplin*. I would also like to thank *P. Osterhammel* and *K. Terkildsen* for permission to use some of their illustrations.

References

Aran, J.: Patterns of human electrocochleographic responses – normal and pathological. J. acoust. Soc. Am. *49:* 112 (1971).

Brown, D.; Shallop, J.: A clinically useful 500 Hz evoked response. Annu. Convention Am Speech/Hearing/Language Ass., Los Angeles 1981.

Davis, H.: Principles of electric response audiometry. Ann. Otol. Rhinol. Lar., suppl. 28, p. 85, 3-part 3 (1976).

Davis, H.; Hirsh, K.: A slow brain stem response for low frequency audiometry. Audiology *18:* 445–461 (1979).

Fria, T.: The auditory brain stem response: background and clinical applications. Monogr. contemp. Audiol., vol. 2 (Maico Hearing Instruments, Minneapolis 1980).

Fria, T.; Kunov, H.; Shallop, J.: School for electric response audiometry. Parts I and II (Madsen Electronics, Toronto 1979).

Galambos, R.; Makeig, S.; Talmachoff, P.: A 40-Hz auditory potential recorded from the human scalp. Proc. natn. Acad. Sci. USA *78:* 2643–2647 (1981).

Jewett, D.; Williston, J.: Auditory-evoked far fields averaged from the scalp of humans. Brain *94:* 681–696 (1971).

Osterhammel, P.; Davis, H.; Weir, C.; Hirsh, S.: Adult auditory evoked vertex potentials in sleep. Audiology *12:* 116–128 (1973).

Picton, T.; Hillyard, S.; Krausz, H.; Galambos, R.: Human auditory evoked potentials. I. Evaluation of components. Electroenceph. clin. Neurophysiol. *36:* 179–190 (1974).

Picton, T.; Woods, D.; Baribeau-Braun, J.: Evoked potential audiometry. Can. J. Otolaryngol. *6:* 90–119 (1977).

Salamy, A.; Mc Kean, C.: Postnatal development of human brainstem potentials during the first year of life. Electroenceph. clin. Neurophysiol. *40:* 418–426 (1976).

Terkildsen, K.; Osterhammel, P.; Huis int Feld, F.: Electrocochleography with a far field technique. Scand. Audiol. *2:* 141–148 (1973).

Worden, F.; Marsh, J.: Frequency-following (microphonic-like) neural responses evoked by sound. Electroenceph. clin. Neurophysiol. *25:* 42–45 (1968).

Yoshie, N.: Auditory nerve action potential responses to clicks in man. Laryngoscope, St. Louis. *78:* 198–214 (1968).

Jon K. Shallop, Ph. D., Department of Otolaryngology and Head and Neck Surgery, Indiana University School of Medicine, Indianapolis, IN 46223 (USA)

Adv. Oto-Rhino-Laryng., vol. 29, pp. 140–144 (Karger, Basel 1983)

Brainstem Electrical Response Audiometry

K. Terkildsen, P. Osterhammel

ENT Department, Rigshospitalet, Copenhagen, Denmark

The primary aim with the development of the auditory brainstem response (ABR) to a clinical tool was to measure hearing objectively in children that for various reasons were untestable and where some kind of sedation was necessary in order to reduce the biological electrical noise that comes with body movements, eye-blinking and so on. It is fair to say that today these problems have been solved. There are several sedation schemes that have been shown to be effective in large series of children, and with modern recording techniques we are now able to resolve response patterns that have a magnitude of only 50–100 nV by means of averaging 1–2000 sweeps. This tells us that the general noise level does not exceed 2–4 μV.

The problems that remain are how to interpret the results and in particular how they relate to conventional audiograms. Ordinarily such discussions are conducted in terms of intensity and specificity with regard to frequency, but as we shall see these parameters are interrelated in a complex manner that only can be understood, if we know the integration time for the ABR, or which part of the stimulus really participates in the generation of a response.

Onishi and Davis [1968] studied these relations for the slow cortical responses and found an integration time of about 30 ms. This agrees with the clinical experience that we with this particular response obtain results that are very comparable to the conventional audiogram. They emphasized the importance of using stimulus envelopes with a linear rise of amplitude. Otherwise the experimental results would be difficult to interpret. With the use of such a linear rise of amplitude the final intensity naturally depends on the duration of the rise-time. If the slope is

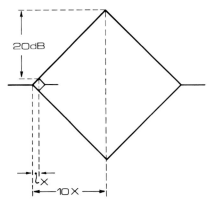

Fig. 1. Schematic illustration of the relation between stimulus duration and final intensity, when the stimulus rise time is linear. Notice that the scale for the ordinate is linear.

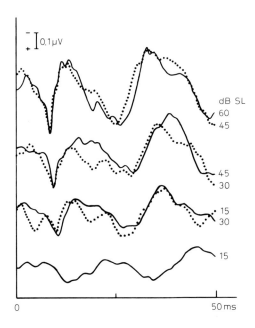

Fig. 2. MLR responses towards 2-kHz tone burst with linear rise of amplitude and different durations as indicated. The slopes for those responses that are superimposed are the same, but due to the different durations the final intensity is not the same. $-$ = 10–0.5–10 ms; ..... 1.5–0.5–1.5 ms.

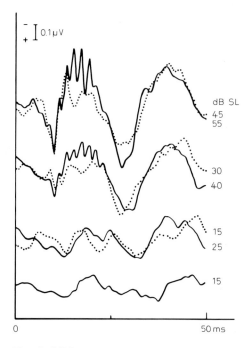

Fig. 3. MLR responses towards 500-Hz tone bursts. — = 10–0.5–10 ms; ..... 3–0.5–3 ms. See text to figure 2.

constant the final intensity increases by 20 dB for each 10-fold increase of duration, and a stimulus that has for instance a rise-time of 15 ms will reach an intensity that is 20 dB stronger than a stimulus that is permitted a rise-time of only 1.5 ms. It is critical to understand this when we compare different stimuli (fig. 1; notice the linear scales both for the X and the Y-axis). If we presume that a response has a very short integration time and that it has been determined already in the course of the first 1.5 ms, then it should remain the same even if the stimulus is permitted to last 15 ms, where it reaches a final intensity that is 20 dB stronger.

Suzuki and Horiuchi [1981] investigated the ABR on the basis of such considerations and found that the integration time at 2 kHz was 1.5 ms or less, and at 500 Hz, 3 ms or less. We have conducted a similar study for the middle latency responses (MLR), and used the same stimuli as *Suzuki and Horiuchi* [1981], 500 and 2,000 Hz. For 2,000 Hz the rise-decay times were 1.5 and 10 ms. With a linear slope the 10-ms sti-

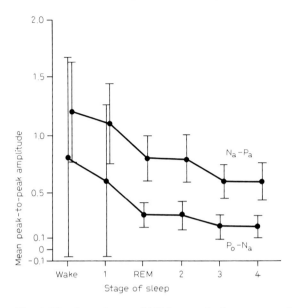

Fig. 4. The dependance of MLR magnitude on stage of sleep [from *Mendel and Goldstein,* 1971].

mulus is 15 dB stronger than the 1.5-ms stimulus, and if this is for instance 50 dB, then the 10-ms stimulus must be 65 dB in order to generate the same amount of stimulation during the initial part of the onset.

The question is now whether the 65 dB, 10-ms lasting stimulus will generate a better response than the shorter and weaker stimulus. Here is an example (fig. 2). The response towards the two types of stimuli have been superimposed and it is quite apparent that there is no difference. This is true also with intensities that are close to the threshold of hearing, and we have not been able to detect any modifications of the response that should be caused by those parts of the stimulus that follows the first 1.5 ms (fig. 3). Here are similar results for the 500-Hz stimulus. The shortest rise-time is 3 ms, which is only 1½ waves up. This is compared with a 10-ms rise-time. With a constant slope the intensity increases close to 10 dB from 3 to 10 ms, so here we compared a 60-dB 10-ms stimulus with a short 50-dB stimulus. At higher intensities the long-lasting stimulus generates a frequency following response which rides on a vertex-negative deviation, but otherwise the responses again are the same.

The stimuli were presented binaurally in order to increase the response magnitude. The bandpass of the filters extended from 30 to 500 Hz with a 24 dB/oct. roll-off at the low end and 12 dB/oct. at the high end. The experiments were conducted on 5 normal subjects and in no one did we find any evidence that those parts of the MLR that extend to the N_b wave have integration times that are longer than those that have been found for wave$_v$ of the ABR. It is quite possible that the integration times are even shorter than the shortest stimuli that were used here and both the ABR and the MLR are on-off responses. When in spite of this we are still able to obtain some degree of frequency specificity with these tests, we believe it can only be explained as a result of cochlear mechanics.

Another consequence is that in normal-hearing individuals the response threshold is about 25 dB poorer than the conventional audiometric threshold, where the stimuli by definition must last at least 200 ms in order to utilize the full integration time for hearing. The MLR is sensitive towards sleep and thus undoubtedly also towards sedation (fig. 4), in spite that it is an on-off type of response with very short integration times, and the prospects for finding responses that are resistant towards sleep and at the same time have longer integration times are indeed dim.

We will have to reconcile ourselved with the fact that although we can measure hearing with the ABR and the MLR, we cannot produce audiograms, and we will have to establish special norms for the results that are obtained with these tests.

References

Mendel, M.; Goldstein, R.: Early components of the averaged electroencephalic response to constant level clicks during all-night sleep. J. Speech Hear. Res. *14:* 829–840 (1971).

Onishi, S.; Davis, H.: Effect of duration and rise time of tone bursts on evoked V potentials. J. acoust. Soc. Am. *44:* 582–592 (1968).

Suzuki, T.; Horiuchi, K.: Rise time of pure-tone stimuli in brain stem response audiometry. Audiology *20:* 101–112 (1981).

K. Terkildsen, MD, ENT Department, Rigshospitalet,
DK-2100 Copenhagen (Denmark)

Adv. Oto-Rhino-Laryng., vol. 29, pp. 145–150 (Karger, Basel 1983)

Ototoxicity of Aminoglycoside Antibiotics in Animal Study

Kiichi Sato

Department of ENT, Kanazawa Medical University, Uchinada, Ishikawa, Japan

Introduction

It is well known that aminoglycoside antibiotics have ototoxicity and induce sensorineural hearing loss. Recently, various kinds of new aminoglycoside antibiotics have been developed. These antibiotics, however, have some degree of ototoxicity. In the terminological conception, ototoxicity is divided into cochlear and vestibular toxicity.

In the clinical feature, the symptoms and signs of ototoxicity are limited to tinnitus, sensorineural hearing loss and depressed vestibular function with or without nystagmus. Characteristic audiograms showed sacrifice of high frequency sensitivity and sometimes total loss in any frequencies. And it is clarified that the primary lesions due to aminoglycoside antibiotics were sensory epithelia of the inner ear by the methods of function test and/or morphological examinations.

In the present paper, the author will explain how the ototoxicity of these antibiotics is evaluated in animals, and also present some interesting results from our animal and clinical studies.

Methodology

The author usually used guinea pigs as experimental animals for ototoxicity, because the cochlea of a guinea pig is protruded in the middle ear cavity without surrounding bony tissue and it has therefore advantages for direct observation and treatment in the experimental procedure. For the evaluation of ototoxicity of aminoglycosides in ani-

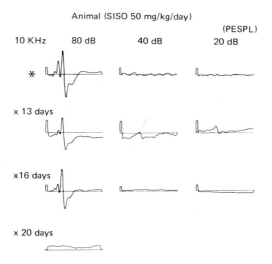

Fig. 1. ABR recording of sisomicin treated animal. The first line (*) showed ABR recording of status before administration, which was limited in 20 dB (arrow). After administration of sisomicin 50 mg/kg for 16 days, the threshold of ABR increased to 80 dB, showing in third line. On 20th day, ABR recording could not be recorded.

mals, there are two methods: one is a functional examination and the other is a morphological examination. By these two methods, cochlear and vestibular toxicities can be examined.

Functional Examination

Regarding the functional test for hearing, the pinna reflex test, cochlear microphonics (CM) and auditory brain response (ABR) are routinely employed. The pinna reflex test is performed to examine changes in hearing sensitivity of animals in response to the pure tone using the differential frequency pinna reflex audiometer (Nagashima Co. Ltd, Japan) and has been applied quite often, as it is a simple method for guinea pigs. This test is considered to be suitable for testing the hearing sensitivity of animals which have received the drug over a long period of time, for no surgical procedures are necessary. CM is also useful but is not considered a simple method because of the necessity for surgical procedures. ABR recordings, using modified Teledyne-Avionics (TA-1000, USA), are the most suitable for getting hearing threshold in guinea pigs under the necessity of anesthesia (fig. 1). The

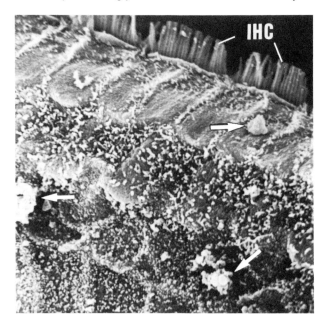

Fig. 2. SEM findings of surface of Corti's organ, showing disappearance of auditory hairs and forming debris (arrow) of outer hair cells after administration of sisomicin 50 mg/kg for 20 days. No remarkable change was present in inner hair cells (IHC). × 3000.

results of ABR recording correlate well with those from the morphological examination (fig. 2).

For the test of equilibrium, the author has employed the righting reflex test and recording of postrotatory electronystagmography (ENG). The former test is a very simple and useful method for screening abnormal condition. Postrotatory ENG recording is a suitable method to evaluate the vestibular function. After administration of drugs, duration of nystagmus is shortened within 3 s and/or disappears (fig. 3). These recordings correspond with degeneration of vestibular epithelia (fig. 4).

Morphological Examination
Regarding the morphological examination, methods of (a) histopathology, (b) histochemistry, (c) transmissional electron microscopy

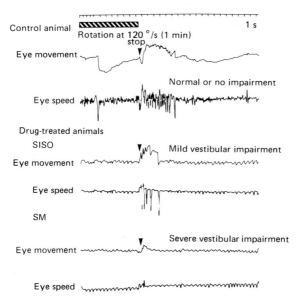

Fig. 3. ENG recordings of postrotatory nystagmus in guinea pigs. Duration of nystagmus in control animals was 5–7 seconds. Duration of nystagmus in mild to moderate damaged animal due to sisomicin was shortened with in about 3 seconds and/or disappeared in severe damaged animal due to streptomycin.

(TEM) and scanning electron microscopy (SEM) are employed. Each of these observations has both advantages and disadvantages.

Histopathological examination has advantages of facility for serial observation, possibility for the observation of the extent of degenerated sensory epithelial cells in cochlea and permanent preservation of specimens. However, a long-term procedure for the specimens is needed. Histochemical examination is performed by the surface preparation technique. This technique is relatively difficult and has the drawback of preserving the enzyme activity on the permanent specimens, but is advantageous in obtaining results rapidly. TEM is indeed suitable for studying the cytoarchitecture of sensory epithelial cells, but it is not satisfactory for observing the extent of damaged cells. SEM is the best method for observing the surface views of sensory epithelial cells, especially deformation of auditory and vestibular sensory hairs due to drugs. However, it is not easy to obtain good specimens (fig. 2, 4).

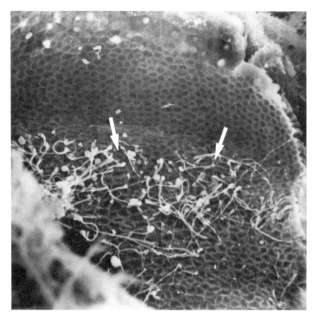

Fig. 4. SEM findings of vestibular sensory hairs of ampullar crista, showing curl-like deformation (arrow) in streptomycin treated animal. × 500.

Degeneration of Sensory Epithelial Cells
Due to Aminoglycoside Antibiotics

It is clarified that sensory epithelial cells of the inner ear have the most sensitive to aminoglycoside antibiotics, especially the outer hair cells in the cochlea and vestibular sensory hair cells of type I. According to SEM observations, auditory hairs of the outer hair cells show the deformation of fan-like spreading, primarily. Then, auditory hairs are changing to fusion, bending and disappearance with protrusion of cuticle of outer hair cells (fig. 2). In the vestibular organ, vestibular sensory hairs took the form of bending (fig. 4), fusion, ballooning, giant hair formation and disappearance on the crista ampullaris, saccular macula and utricular macula. Degeneration of the otoconia is also seen in some animals, which is clearly different from the normal appearance of otoconia.

The author intended to reevaluate the general tendency in the pattern of outer hair cell and inner hair cell loss of Corti's organ in the ototoxicity due to antibiotics by histopathology [*Akiyoshi* et al., 1971] and SEM [*Sato,* 1970, 1980, 1982]. As a result of reevaluation, loss of the outer hair cell always started at the basal end of Corti's organ and then spread upwards. Also, the outer hair cells were more sensitive in the basal and second turns, while the inner hair cell was more sensitive in the apical and fourth turns. In the vestibular organ, vestibular sensory hair cell of type I on the crista ampullaris was more sensitive among the other vestibular sensory hair cells [*Sato,* 1979, 1981]. These tendencies are useful for understanding that sensorineural hearing loss due to aminoglycoside antibiotics occurs in high frequency of audiogram.

References

1   Akiyoshi, M.; Sato, K.; Shoji, T.; Sugahiro, K.: Pattern of hair cell damage of the organ of Corti due to ototoxic antibiotics (in Japanese). Audiol. Jap. *14:* 530–541 (1971).
2   Sato, K.; Koeda, T.; Yokoda, M.: Evaluation of ototoxicity of aminoglycoside antibiotics in guinea pigs by scanning electron microscopy. Curr. Chemother. infect. Dis. *1980:* 608–609.
3   Sato, K.: Ototoxicidad y antibioticos aminoglucosidos. Simp. Sobre Ribostamycin, Lima, 1980, pp. 1–13.
4   Sato, K.; Saito, T.: Comparative study on vestibular toxicity of dibekacin, ribostamycin and other aminoglycoside antibiotics in guinea pig by scanning electron microscopy. Int. J. clin. Pharm. Ther. Tox. *20*(in press, 1982).

K. Sato, MD, Department of ENT, Kanazawa Medical University, Uchinada, Ishikawa 920-02 (Japan)

Adv. Oto-Rhino-Laryng., vol. 29, pp. 151–162 (Karger, Basel 1983)

Otosclerosis, a Universal Disease

Ole Bentzen

Hearing Clinic, Århus Kommunehospitals, Århus, Denmark

In histopathological studies of the otosclerotic process, the discussion whether this is equal to or different from the process in the middle ear in patients with osteogenesis imperfecta, had, through many years, taken place. This study is based on the clinical picture of patients with otosclerosis. Does the clinical examination of these patients support the thesis that otosclerosis, being a hereditable disease, is a part of the group of hereditable disorders of connective tissue? Since 1954 the clinical study of our patients with otosclerosis had demonstrated clinical manifestations equal to those in patients with other hereditable disorders of connective tissue. As a consequence, skin biopsies were taken which through light microscopical examinations showed metachromasia of the ground substance and degeneration of the collagen and elastic fibers [*Bentzen,* 1961]. These findings support the aforementioned thesis that the defective hearing in otosclerosis is but a single manifestation of a generalized disturbance of the organ of connective tissue.

Pathological Studies of the Skin in Patients with Hearing Defects

The first pathological study of skin in patients with hearing defects was performed by *Follis* [1952]. He called attention to certain hitherto unreported morphological alterations in the skin, eye and skeletal tissue of an infant coming to autopsy with the classical manifestations of osteogenesis imperfecta. In 1961, *Stadil,* in a study of skin biopsies from patients with osteogenesis imperfecta, from our clinic, found exactly the same picture as we had in patients with otosclerosis. Tissue biopsies from the middle ear of patients operated for otosclerosis have been examined by *Oglivie and Hall* [1953] resulting in the suggestion by these authors that otosclerosis was related to a general affection of mesenchym. This thesis was supported by *Arslan and Ricci* [1960] by histochemical examination of the tissue from the middle ear of these patients. Microscopical examination of the vessels of the facial skin [*Vyslonzil,* 1956] and skin samples of the external acoustic canal of 54 patients with otosclerosis [*Pavlov* et al., 1981] concludes that this disease might formally have a collagenous character.

Biochemical investigations of vein tissue taken from patients with otosclerosis had demonstrated that the average lactic dehydrogenase activity in vein tissue from 81 of these patients was 30% higher than the average activity observed in vein tissue from 40 normal persons. *Soifer* et al. [1965] therefore conclude that their report supports the premise that otosclerosis is associated with a general disorder. In our clinical examination of patients with this disease we found abnormalities in the organs derived from the ectoderm (skin, nails and hair) and from the mesoderm (joints, teeth and vessels) indicating the existence of an ectomesodermal insufficiency (EMI). In order to find an atraumatic objective method for the diagnosis of EMI, *Ehlers,* Head of the Ophthalmological Department, University Hospital, Århus, suggested the use of corneometry which is a method of measuring the thickness of the central part of the cornea.

Ophthalmological Studies

In 1903, *Buchanan* [quoted after *Ruedemann,* 1903] studied the eye of a 9-year-old girl whose eye required enucleation because of an injury. Blue sclerotics were a family trait, but bone defects were not noted in the child or in her family. Ophthalmological examination revealed myopia and conical cornea. On histological examination a diminished number of scleral fibers and cells were noted. The cornea was similarly defective. In a study by *Ruedemann* [1953], 3 cases of osteogenesis imperfecta are reported. In the prescription of the ocular pathology, the author concludes that the abnormalities in the fibrous coats of the eye – especially the corneal stroma and the sclerae – would appear to be similar to the changes in the bone and skin, namely deficiency in collagen formation. In order to look for the same phenomenon in spontaneous retinal detachment, central corneal thickness in these patients was studied [*Kruse Hansen* et al., 1971]. Corneometry was performed in 40 consecutively operated cases of retinal detachment. Central corneal thickness was found to be significantly lower than normal in detachment eyes as well as in contralateral eyes. Histological examination of skin biopsies from 17 of the patients revealed a smaller thickness of epidermis and degenerative changes in collagenous and elastic fibers. The results suggest a universal abnormality of constitution, possibly as a predisposition to development of retinal detachment.

Corneometry in Patients with Hearing Defects

By using the Haag-Streit pachymeter, modified by *Ehlers and Sperling* [1977], the thickness of the cornea can be measured in an optical way. The normal values are between 0.475 and 0.535 mm. The results are plotted in a corneogram where the triangle at the bottom covers the normal values. Individuals with either thin or thick cornea are indicated as cornea-positive, those with normal values cornea-negative.

Since 1965, patients with otosclerosis have been tested by corneometry either done at the Eye Department or, since May 1979, by the Haag-Streit pachymeter at the Audiological Clinic where this examination is part of the routine for all patient groups. Dr. *Groes* examines patients with hearing defects, patients with other diseases and normal individuals. Corneometry examination of an increasing number of individuals is performed in order to clarify the thesis that cornea positivity is an important factor in the determination of EMI.

Cornea Positivity and Its Somatic Relations

The study of its relation to *chromosomes* had been made in collaboration with *Henriksen and Ehlers* [1972] as a part of a large-scale investigation on male, juvenile criminals. In 98 cases, all examined by corneometry, analysis of the chromosomes had been done at the Cytogenetic Institute by *Nielsen*, Head of the Department of Psychiatry, University of Århus. 9 cases with abnormal chromosomes are plotted in the corneogram shown in figure 1. 1 case had a thin cornea and 2 had a thick one. 1 of these (No. 62) had Klinefelter's syndrome 47XXY.

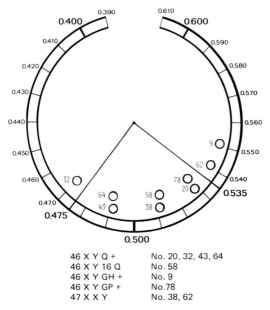

Fig. 1. Corneogram with the distribution of 9 cases of abnormal chromosome.

Table I. Corneometry and type B27

Disease	Total	Cornea-positive	Cornea-negative	
Plus B27				
Morbus Reiter	6	3	3	
Other	13	8	5	11/19
Minus B27				
Morbus Reiter	5	0	5	
Other	7	2	5	2/12

Thickness of cornea in 31 patients from the Department of Rheumatology, University Hospital, Århus 1981: of 13 cornea-positive patients 11 had type B27.

Among the 89 persons with normal chromosomes, 23 were cornea-positive (7 thin, 16 thick). The 30% cornea-positive among the abnormal chromosome cases versus 25% among the normal cases do not show any significant distribution. The same results are found in the material of corneometry in mongoloid children and their parents.

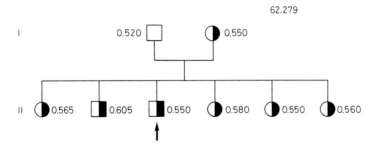

Fig. 2. Family A: the proband is indicated by the arrow. The values of corneometry indicated in figures.

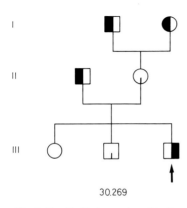

Fig. 3. Family B: the proband indicated by the arrow showed a thick cornea and the 3 cornea-positive members a thin cornea.

Cornea-positive cases in relation to the HLA system are studied in patients treated at the rheumatological department at the hospital, where corneometry and determination of HLA-B27 had been performed. The relation between patients with plus-B27 and minus-B27, both groups divided into those with morbus Reiter and those with other rheumatological diseases is shown in table I. Among 19 plus-B27 patients, 11 were cornea-positive in contrast to only 2 patients in the minus-B27 group [*Jurik*, pers. commun.].

The occurrence of abnormal thickness of cornea in families, i.e. the *genetic appearance* had been studied in some families from which families A and B are selected as examples.

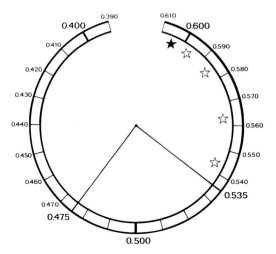

Fig. 4. The values of corneometry of the blind mother (★) and her 4 normal children (☆) plotted in a corneogram.

Case 62.279

Male, born 1953. The mother's father and mother had been hard of hearing since 30 years of age. The brother had bilateral high tone loss as found in his sisters (No. 3 and 4). The cornea thickness values are indicated in the family tree (fig. 2). The genetic rules are still unsolved. In family A, all cornea-positive cases have thick cornea. In family B there is a change over from generations I and II to generation III. Observations similar to these have been seen in other family trees.

Case 30.269

Male, born 1965, birth weight 4 kg, had a very severe bilateral sensorineural hearing defect. During pregnancy the mother was infected by rubella. Her parents were both cornea-positive (0.460 mm). Both the mother (0.485 mm) and brother (0.510 mm) were normal. The father (0.460 mm) and the boy himself (0.550 mm) were both cornea-positive (fig. 3).

Cornea positivity in individuals with *pathological skin biopsies:* this is illustrated in the aforementioned study of patients with retinal detachment and in a case history.

Case 63.107

Female, born 1931, at the age of 45 and within a period of 8 months developed bilateral optic neuritis causing blindness. Corneometry showed 0.605 mm. Light microscopical examination of the skin showed atrophy of the epidermis and degenerative changes in the collagen and elastic fibers.

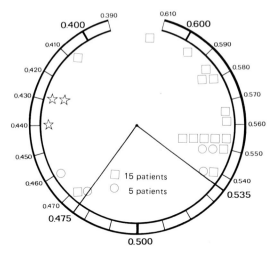

Fig. 5. Corneogram with different types of otosclerosis and 3 cases of osteogenesis imperfecta. ☆ = Osteogenesis imperfecta; ○ = otosclerosis cochlearis; □ = otosclerosis, other types.

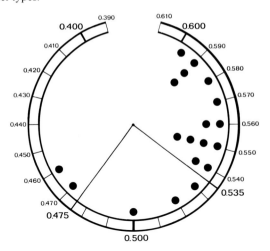

Fig. 6. Distribution of corneometry in 19 women with sensorineural hearing loss, all X-ray-positive by polytomography of os temporale (●).

All 4 children were examined: daughter (19 years) corneometry 0.600 mm; son (28 years) corneometry 0.585 mm; daughter (15 years) corneometry 0.565 mm; daughter (30 years) corneometry 0.545 mm. All were healthy. Examination of the skin in all 4 children showed mild degenerative abnormalities of the collagen fibers. All 5 indicated in figure 4 had normal hearing.

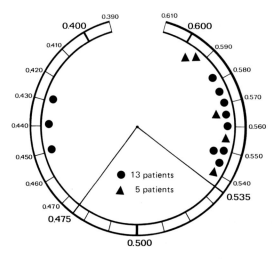

Fig. 7. The distribution of the results of corneometry in 12 cases of nontraumatic (●) and 10 cases of noise traumatic perceptive hearing loss (▲).

The relation of abnormal thickness of the cornea and *hearing defects in otosclerosis* is the main goal in the project and is only shown in some examples. The corneogram (fig. 5) shows some of the early analysis of patients with different types of otosclerosis compared with findings in cases of osteogenesis imperfecta. A great deal of material has been published by *Bramsen and Pedersen* [1980] on this syndrome. Thin cornea was demonstrated in a group of 22 patients, the average thickness being 0.427 ± 0.004 mm. In this material, 14 patients had a hearing loss.

The distribution of cornea-positive versus negative cases in the different types of otosclerosis is rather uncharacteristic as shown in figure 5. Therefore, a detailed study of cochlear otosclerosis was performed in 132 patients with sensorineural hearing defects. Polytomography was done in the semiaxial and axial pyramidal projections in all patients [*Sindrason* et al. 1975]. In all, 72 patients showed different degrees of sclerotic abnormalities on the X-ray film. Of these patients, 38 (19 women, 19 men) had been called upon for corneometry. Of the 23 patients, 7 men and 16 of the 19 women were cornea-positive. The distribution of the corneal values in the female material is plotted in a corneogram (fig. 6). This result using *Valvassori's* polytomography technique is in accordance with the technique used by *Linthicum* who in 111 individuals with progressive sensorineural hearing loss of 40 dB or more found 77 X-ray-positive patients with evidence of otosclerotic foci by polytomography. More details about the diagnosis of cochlear otosclerosis are to be found in a paper by *Shaumbaugh* [1973]. In order to explore the value of corneometry in finding persons at risk of *noise deafness* this method is routinely used in patients with sensorineural hearing defects. One of our first series is shown in a corneogram (fig. 7).

In 1961, *Bentzen and Stadil* published 2 cases of acute bilateral noise trauma where biopsy of the skin had shown exactly the same abnormalities as in patients with otosclerosis, patients with retinal detachment and in the 5 persons in case history 63.107. The case history is described of 1 of the noise trauma cases included in figure 7.

Case 63.373

Female, born 1929, a school dentist, working for the last 20 years with aerotor. Repeated checkups of her hearing by audiometry through all the years had shown an increasing bilateral noise deafness. A large group of her colleagues had also been working for a number of years with aerotor without any damage to their hearing. Corneometry showed that she was positive: 0.565 mm. The result of corneometry, in this case history, is in accordance with the clinical observation that this dentist represents a case with decreased resistance to acoustic trauma, as stated by *Bentzen* [1981].

In collaboration with medical doctors in the military services, corneometry was introduced in order to try to evaluate the noise-risk persons as mentioned in case history family A, case 62.279. The results so far seem to indicate that this objective method may be valuable in preoperative selection of soldiers with hearing organs sensitive to noise. In cornea-positive soldiers there seems to be a tendency for the development of a broader dip than in their cornea-negative comrades [*Bundgaard*, pers. commun.]. The occurrence of affection of cornea is evident in many different *hereditable connective tissue syndromes*.

In the literature, genetic hearing loss is published in 125 different syndromes [*Konigsmark and Gorling*, 1976] where sensorineural conductive or mixed hearing loss can occur. Among them, 25 syndromes are associated with eye disease, 13 of which the corneal organ has been affected. Nowhere in the above-mentioned reports is the measurement of the cornea mentioned.

Moestrup [1969] demonstrated severely reduced corneal thickness in Ehlers-Danlos syndrome. In patients with juvenile diabetes, the gen-

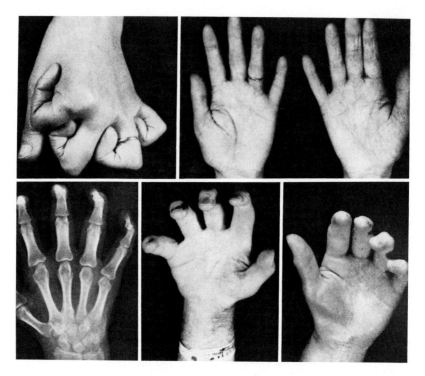

Fig. 8. Top: 37-year-old white female with Ehlers-Danlos syndrome. Bottom: the X-ray and the hand of a 49-year-old white man and hand of his 36-year-old-sister, both representing mucopolysaccharidosis (Scheie syndrome). Apart from their claw hands they both have corneal clouding and the brother sensorineural hearing loss since 37 years of age [from *McKusick* 1965, pp. 198, 369].

etic form of this disease [*Olsen* et al., 1980] from the Eye Department had reported increased thickness of the cornea. Several different cases of syndromes had been examined at the hearing clinic. It is quite evident that the occurrence of thin and thick cornea may occur in the same clinical syndrome.

The Specificity of the Values of the Thickness of Cornea

In 15 cases of identical twins examined so far, the values of the thickness of the cornea were nearly identical. In the literature describing syndromes of hereditable connective tissue disease [*McKusick,*

1965], especially as far as the case histories are concerned, it is quite obvious that both sides of normality are equally important as indicators for abnormality. In syndromes with dysfunction of the sweat glands, hyperhidrosis can be observed in the right arm and hypohidrosis in the left arm of the same patient. Hyperflexibility of the joints, especially the basic joint of the fingers, is often found in these diseases. *Ellis and Bundick* [1956] called the attention to this fact and recommended measurement of the little finger angle as a measure of joint mobility and tissue elasticity. Figure 8 shows the mobility of the fingers in two different syndromes of hereditable disorders of connective tissue. Why should this abnormality on both sides of the normal values not occur in the organ of cornea? There may exist a possibility that the thin cornea seems to occur with a greater frequency in the more generalized affection of the connective tissue, but the problem is not yet solved.

Conclusion

Since 1953, when *Oglivie and Hall* introduced the idea that otosclerosis could be considered as a disease of the collagen, an increasing material on clinical, histological and biochemical data has been published. Introduction of the atraumatic objective method, of studying ectomesodermal insufficiency, by corneometry, had in the audiological clinic to a great extent increased the number of examined individuals. Since 1979, this method, being part of our daily routine, has increased the diagnostic procedures. Experience has shown a high incidence of cornea-positivity in X-ray-positive cases of cochlear otosclerosis. Studies are in development concerning corneometry as in indicator of decreased resistance of the hearing organ to acoustic trauma. Cornea-positive individuals are recognized among persons with normal hearing.

In the HLA system, individuals with plus B27 are very often cornea-positive. This distribution within the chromosome system is still unsolved. From studies of other hereditable diseases of connective tissue it is demonstrated that either thin or thick corneas indicate suspicion of ectomesodermal insufficiency.

The introduction of corneometry in patients with otosclerosis has supported the idea that it is a disease of the collagen. The aforementioned thesis should cover other causes of hearing loss and normal hearing individuals suspected as risk persons in regard to infections. The method of measuring the delicate structure of the organ of cornea, in such a simple way as by corneometry, gives us the possibility of dividing humans into two groups: cornea-negative and cornea-positive. In the whole population, as far as Caucasians are concerned, the cornea-positive individual seems to represent 10% in all.

References

Arslan, M.; Ricci, V.: Oto-rino-lar. ital. *29:* 6 (1960).

Bentzen, O.: Excerpta Med. Int. Congr. Ser., No. 35, abstr. 80, 40 (1961).

Bentzen, O.: Sensorineural hearing loss and somatic insufficiency. Audiology *21:* 97–110 (1982).

Bentzen, O.; Stadil, P.: Ugeskr. Læg. *123:* 663 (1961).

Bramsen, T.; Pedersen, U.: Ugeskr. Læg. *142:* 1609 (1980).

Ehlers, N.; Sperling, S.: Acta ophthal. *55:* 333 (1977).

Ellis, F.E.; Bundick, W.R.: Archs. Derm. *24:* 22 (1956).

Follis, R.H., Jr.: J. Pediat. *41:* 713 (1952).

Konigsmark, B.W.; Gorling, R.J.: Genetic and metabolic deafness (Saunders, Philadelphia 1976).

Kruse Hansen, F.; Ehlers, N.; Bentzen, O.; Søgaard, H.: Acta ophthal. *49:* 467 (1971).

McKusick, V.A.: Heritable disorders of connective tissue (Mosby, St. Louis 1965).

Moestrup, B.: Acta ophthal. *47:* 704 (1969).

Oglivie, R.F.; Hall, I.S.: J. Laryng. *67:* 497 (1953).

Olsen, T.; Busted, N.; Schmitz, O.: Lancet *i:* 80 (1980).

Pavlov, V.; Fitscheva, M.; Zenev, I.: HNO-Praxis, Leipzig *6:* 12 (1981).

Ruedemann, A.D., Jr.: Archs Ophthal. *49:* 6 (1953).

Shaumbaugh, G.E.: Archs Otolar. *97:* 30 (1973).

Sindrason, E.; Eriksen, P.O.; Halaburt, H.: Læknabladid *65:* 91 (1975).

Soifer, N.; Altmann, F.; Endahl, G.L.; Holdswoth, C.: Archs Otolar. *82:* 510 (1965).

Stadil, P.: Excerpta Med. Int. Congr. Ser., No. 35, abstr. 331, 124 (1961).

Vyslonzil, E.Z.: Lar. Rhinol. Otol. *35:* 185 (1956).

O. Bentzen, MD, Hearing Clinic, Århus Kommunehospitals,
DK-8000 Århus (Denmark)

Adv. Oto-Rhino-Laryng., vol. 29, pp. 163–173 (Karger, Basel 1983)

Loudness of Tinnitus:
An Approach to Measurement

R. Hinchcliffe, Christine Chambers

Institute of Laryngology and Otology, London, England

Introduction

In the study of tinnitus it is frequently desirable to assess how loud the sound (or sounds) appears to the afflicted individual. The measurement of loudness owes much to the work of *Stevens* [1955] and his collaborators. Although these studies apply to external sounds they may be equally well applicable to internal sounds.

Stevens [1955] showed that the Weber-Fechner logarithmic function was invalid and that a power function gave a better fit to the available data:

$$\Psi = k\Phi^n, \tag{1}$$

where Ψ = psychological magnitude of stimulus, Φ = physical magnitude of stimulus, k = a constant, and n = a constant.

Subsequently, *Scharf and Stevens* [1959] showed that a more appropriate psychophysical relationship was obtained by subtracting the physical magnitude of the physiological zero from the physical magnitude of the relevant stimulus,

$$\Psi = k(\Phi - \Phi_0)^n, \tag{2}$$

where Ψ = psychological magnitude of stimulus, Φ = physical magnitude of stimulus, Φ_0 = physical magnitude of threshold stimulus, k = a constant, and n = a constant.

Lochner and Burger [1961] have claimed that low intensity data are better fitted by the equation:

$$\Psi = k(\Phi^n - \Phi_0^n), \tag{3}$$

where Ψ = psychological magnitude of stimulus, Φ = physical magnitude of stimulus, Φ_0 = physical magnitude of threshold stimulus, k = a constant, and n = a constant.

It would appear that it should be possible, following an intensity matching of tinnitus, to specify its loudness in sones (the unit of loudness). Since the sone is defined as the loudness of a pure tone at a frequency of 1 kHz and at a sound level of 40 dB SPL the appropriate procedure is to match the tinnitus to a 1-kHz tone. This binaural loudness match is thus also a bifrequency match.

Whilst this binaural bifrequency match is a relatively simple procedure using Békésy type audiometry, the problem of interindividual differences remains. A noise with a calculated loudness of 1 sone may not seem to be the same loudness to two different people. Moreover, a sound that is equally loud to two different individuals may be acceptable to one but not to the other.

The purpose of this pilot study, therefore, was to assess to what extent one could construct individual psychophysical functions in the clinical situation, and which functions would reflect not only individual differences in the growth of loudness but also individual differences in loudness acceptability.

Method

9 consecutive patients who had continual, unilateral tinnitus and who were able to match their tinnitus to a pure tone were studied. 7 subjects, who were drawn from the staff of the Institute of Laryngology and Otology where the study was conducted, and who were matched as far as possible for age and sex, served as controls. The age range of the tinnitus patients ranged from 15 to 79 years; that of the control group 18–50 years.

The patients had been subjected to an intensive neuro-otological investigation.

Using a Békésy-type audiometer in the pulsed test tone mode, the following measurements were performed on the ear contralateral to the tinnitus in each patient: (1) pitch match of the tinnitus; (2) loudness match of the tinnitus using a pure tone of a frequency which had been matched to the pitch of the tinnitus; (3) threshold of hearing at 1 kHz; (4) loudness match of tinnitus to a tone of 1 kHz; (5) repeat threshold at 1 kHz; (6) most comfortable loudness level at 1 kHz; (7) repeat threshold at 1 kHz; (8) loudness level at 1 kHz which was judged by the subject to be half as loud as the loudness of the tone at the most comfortable loudness level; (9) repeat threshold at 1 kHz; (10) loudness level at 1 kHz which was judged by the subject to be twice as loud as the loudness of the sound at the most comfortable loudness level; (11) repeat threshold at 1 kHz; (12) the level of a 1 kHz tone which was at the threshold of uncomfortable loudness. The subject was also asked to assign a number to this loudness which would indicate how much louder this tone was than one at the most comfortable loudness level.

The last eight measurements were also performed on the control subjects. 1 control subject was also tested on two additional occasions to explore the degree of intraindividual variability.

The various loudness levels were tabulated for each subject. Using the data for each individual, attempts were made to calculate the best-fit equation for *Scharf and Stevens'* [1959] power function and *Lochner and Burger's* [1961] power function. The criterion adopted for the equation of best fit in the latter case was considered to be when the intercept in the following equation was zero:

$$\Psi = k(\Phi^n - \Phi_0^n) + b \tag{4}$$

Finding the solution was facilitated using an iterative procedure on a microcomputer.

Results

The statistical analysis of the data showed that neither age nor sex influenced the results.

Tables I and II show the measured most comfortable loudness levels for the subjects in the control and the tinnitus groups, respectively. The most comfortable loudness level for each subject is shown in the fourth column (M) of the tables. These measurements, as well as the other measurements given in tables I and II, are expressed in dB HL. The hearing levels corresponding to half and twice the loudness of that of the most comfortable loudness level are given in the third and fifth columns, respectively. The thresholds of uncomfortable loudness (TUL) are given in the final column. The number in parenthesis which immediately follows the TUL is the loudness magnitude (MCLL as unity) which was assigned by the subject to the tone at the TUL.

For the control group and the tinnitus group respectively, tables III and IV show the constants in the calculated best fit power functions for the equation given by *Scharf and Stevens* [1959] (the exponent, n, and the scaling factor, k, are shown in the second and third columns respectively). The final column shows the product moment correlation coefficient. With this sample size, a coefficient of 0.95 is significant at the $p < 0.05$ level, of 0.990 at the $p < 0.01$ level, and of 0.999 at the $p < 0.001$ level.

Tables V and VI show similar values to those listed in tables III and IV except that these are derived for the best fit equation to Lochner and Burger's power function.

Illustrations to show the goodness of fit of a power function of the Scharf and Stevens' type are shown in figures 1–5. Figures 1–3 are from control subjects, figures 4 and 5 are from patients with tinnitus. Figures

Table I. Controls

Subject	Threshold	0.5 M	M	2 M	TUL
A.R.N.	4	33	54	62	71 (4)
H.A.N.	2	51	67	82	95 (3)
K.A.V.	6	42	62	73	87 (3)
K.E.N.	19	47	60	92	95 (4)
L.I.L.	15	36	49	59	76 (4)
M.A.K.	–4	31	57	84	87 (2)
P.O.M.	1	67	76	83	97 (4)
Median	4	42	60	82	87 (4)

Values for the threshold, loudness corresponding to half that of the most comfortable loudness level (0.5 M), the most comfortable loudness level (M), the loudness corresponding to twice that of the most comfortable loudness level (2 M) and the threshold of uncomfortable loudness (TUL) expressed in dB HL. The final value in parentheses is the subjective magnitude of the loudness of the TUL as a multiple of the loudness of the most comfortable loudness level.

Table II. Tinnitus group

Subject	Threshold	0.5 M	M	2 M	TUL
A.C.Q.	36	56	64	92	101 (3)
A.R.A.	1	34	52	59	61 (2)
B.A.N.	5	21	27	40	42 (2)
B.O.W.	7	15	43	73	87 (2)
B.R.A.	26	32	36	66	52 (2)
H.Y.N.	1	17	32	56	91 (4)
M.I.T.	16	47	56	78	88 (4)
S.A.N.	18	24	42	50	48 (1.5)
S.H.A.	44	61	72	101	103 (2)
Median	16	32	43	66	87 (2)

See table I for explanations.

Table III. Best fit Scharf and Stevens' function: controls

Subject	Exponent (n)	k	R
A.R.N.	0.41	5.99	0.981
H.A.N.	0.36	2.28	0.997
K.A.V.	0.36	3.12	0.992
K.E.N.	0.31	2.30	0.958
L.I.L.	0.45	7.52	0.995
M.A.K.	0.22	2.08	0.999
P.O.M.	0.61	2.19	0.989
Median	0.36	2.30	0.992

Values of the calculated exponent, scaling factor (k) and product moment correlation coefficient (R) for the best fit Scharf and Stevens' power function.

Table IV. Best fit Scharf and Stevens' function: tinnitus group

Subject	Exponent (n)	k	R
A.C.Q.	0.304	1.81	0.977
A.R.A.	0.455	7.65	0.977
B.A.N.	0.525	33.25	0.981
B.O.W.	0.167	2.27	0.985
B.R.A.	0.286	4.95	0.910
H.Y.N.	0.234	3.97	0.986
M.I.T.	0.401	3.53	0.986
S.A.N.	0.346	7.40	0.967
S.H.A.	0.261	1.31	0.977
Median	0.304	3.97	0.977

See table III for explanations.

Table V. Fitted Lochner and Burger function: controls

Subject	Exponent (n)	k	R
A.R.N.	0.42	6.70	0.988
H.A.N.	0.32	2.35	0.997
K.A.V.	0.31	3.22	0.990
K.E.N.	0.26	2.81	0.893
L.I.L.	0.35	6.88	0.997
M.A.K.	0.13	2.77	0.997
S.O.M.	0.54	2.19	0.992
Median	0.32	2.81	0.992

See table III for explanations.

Table VI. Fitted Lochner and Burger functions: tinnitus group

Subject	Exponent (n)	k	R
A.C.Q.	0.15	3.31	0.985
A.R.A.	0.47	8.66	0.973
B.A.N.	0.32	14.78	0.989
B.O.W.	*	*	*
B.R.A.	*	*	*
H.Y.N.	0.08	6.84	1.000
M.I.T.	0.38	3.78	0.984
S.A.N.	*	*	*
S.H.A.	0.02	13.00	0.997
Median	0.08		

See table III for explanations.
* Exponent $< 1 \times 10^{-6}$.

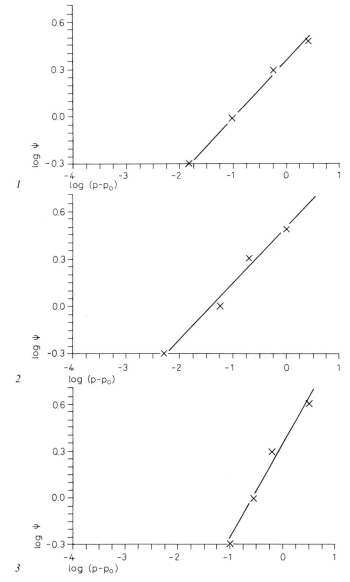

Fig. 1. Results for subject H.A.N. expressed on logarithmic coordinates. Control subject.

Fig. 2. Results for subject C.A.V. expressed on logarithmic coordinates. Control subject.

Fig. 3. Results for subject P.O.M. expressed on logarithmic coordinates. Control subject.

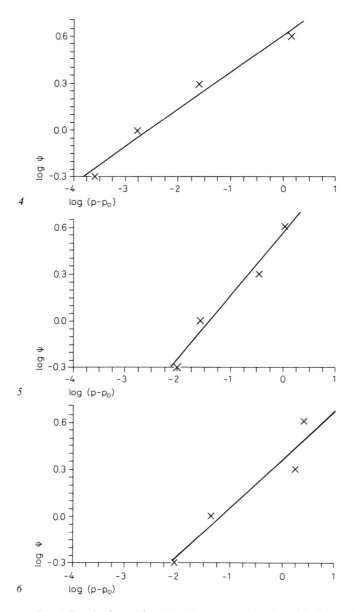

Fig. 4. Results for subject H.Y.N. expressed on logarithmic coordinates. Subject with tinnitus.

Fig. 5. Results for subject M.I.T. expressed on logarithmic coordinates. Subject with tinnitus.

Fig. 6. Results for subject K.E.N. on the first occasion.

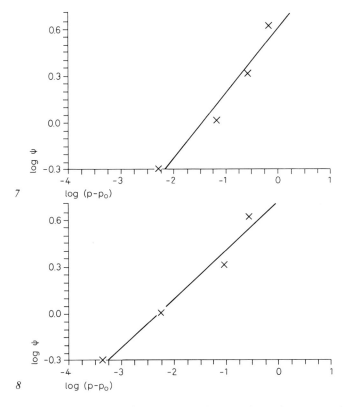

Fig. 7. Results for subject K.E.N. on the second occasion.
Fig. 8. Results for subject K.E.N. on the third occasion.

6–8 show the plots for the data obtained when a single subject was tested three times at intervals of about a week.

An analysis of the data failed to demonstrate that either the exponents or the scaling factors were significantly correlated with the
threshold of hearing.

Discussion

This method of constructing an individual loudness function in
clinical practice is shown to be a feasible procedure when calculations
are based upon Scharf and Stevens' psychophysical function. As table

VI indicates, a construction based on the Lochner and Burger function is not possible in many cases.

With this procedure, unit loudness for a given subject has been defined as that loudness which corresponds to the loudness of a 1-kHz tone which the subject judges to be at his most comfortable loudness level. To distinguish these loudness units from sones, they could be referred to as PLU (personal loudness units). These units have the advantage over sones in that they reflect personal differences in the growth of the loudness function and relate loudness to what might be termed the optimum loudness for a given subject, i.e. his MCLL.

A point of particular interest is that the rate of growth of loudness, as measured by this procedure, is almost half of that of the sone scale. Further studies are therefore required to elucidate this discrepancy. The different growth rates do not seem to arise because of the presence of tinnitus since similar exponents were exhibited by the control group.

Additional studies are also required to elucidate the factors which determine the rate of growth of loudness, as measured by this procedure. There is a large variability. For a control group, and in regard to the exponent, n, in the best fitted Scharf and Stevens' equation, the coefficient of variation is 31%; for the tinnitus group, it is 34%. The scaling factor, k, shows even greater variability. The coefficient of variation for the corresponding two groups is 50 and 135%. As figures 6–8 show, some of this variability is accounted for by intrasubject variability, but it would appear that a large intersubject variability still remains. Analysis of this data failed to show a correlation with auditory threshold. Because of the influence of loudness recruitment, one would expect to find that the exponent would be inversely related to threshold. The study of larger samples with different types of hearing impairment is clearly indicated.

As shown in tables I and II, tinnitus patients have a lower MCLL than apparently otologically normal subjects. This is not primarily due to the phenomenon of loudness recruitment since this finding is observed when the measurements are expressed in terms of hearing level, and not sensation level. The effect is appreciable. It will be noted that the median MCLL of the tinnitus group is 17 dB less than that of the controls. Although the median threshold of uncomfortable loudness (TUL) is the same for the two groups, the mean TUL is 12 dB less for the tinnitus group. This difference in MCLLs is reflected within the greater scaling factor, k, for the tinnitus group.

Conclusions

Using Békésy-type audiometry, and with concepts of loudness derived from psychoacoustics, it should be possible to determine the loudness of tinnitus in the clinical situation. The methods described in this paper will be suitable for studies of tinnitus in clinical practice. However, further studies are indicated for a number of reasons but, particularly, since the rate of growth of loudness as measured by this method was about half that reported from ratio scaling techniques.

References

Lochner, J.P.A.; Burger, J.F.: Form of the loudness function in the presence of masking noise. J. acoust. Soc. am. *33:* 1705–1707 (1961).

Scharf, B.; Stevens, J.C.: The form of the loudness function near threshold. Proc. 3rd Int. Congr. Acoustics, Stuttgart 1959.

Stevens, S.S.: The measurement of loudness. J. Acoust. Soc. Am. *27:* 815–829 (1955).

R. Hinchcliffe, MD, Institute of Laryngology and Otology, 330 Gray's Inn Road, London WC 1X 8EE (England)

Adv. Oto-Rhino-Laryng., vol. 29, pp. 174–182 (Karger, Basel 1983)

Deafness as a World Problem

Christopher Holborow

Commonwealth Society for the Deaf and Westminster Hospital, London, England

It may be that because otologists spend so much time looking through their operating microscopes they become rather short-sighted and fail to see the wider problems of deafness. It is certainly appropriate during The International Year of the Disabled Person to examine this 'hidden handicap' as a world problem. In order to consider what are the best practical measures to help the deaf and to ensure that deafness receives the attention its severity as a disability warrants, I think we should ask ourselves three questions: (1) How many deaf people are there in the world? What is the extent of the problem? (2) What can we usefully do to help the many – not only the few? The greatest problems are with the rural underprivileged majority rather than the urban minority. (3) What of the future?

I will try briefly to discuss these questions illustrating some of my comments by using figures from a survey *Martinson* and I undertook in Nigeria during the last 3 years.

The World Population

Between 1930 and 1975 the world population has increased by 2,000 million people and has doubled. Today the total is about 4,500 million and the graph is rising. Looking at the population distribution figures (table I) it would seem likely that at least two thirds of the total live in the underprivileged countries and, indeed, the United Nations estimated that in 1979 (The International Year of the Child) that 350 million children were living in conditions where the standards for

Table I. Population of continents of the world

Populations	1975 figures (in millions)
Europe	473
Asia	2,256
USSR	255
Africa	401
America	561
Oceania	21

Table II. International Year of the Child (1979)

Estimated that 350 million children have standards that are below the minimum in:

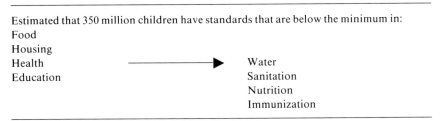

Food
Housing
Health
Education

Water
Sanitation
Nutrition
Immunization

food, housing, education and health were below the acceptable minimum (table II). Taking the customary figure of one profoundly deaf person in every thousand – and it is interesting to note that this figure has never been seriously faulted – there are 4.5 million profoundly deaf people in the world. There are probably 180 million partially deaf. Of this total there are 2 million profoundly deaf children, one sixth of whom are already severely disadvantaged by other causes.

The problems of multiple disability – and deafness is by no means the least component though it may be the least noticed – are compounded by the distribution of medical care in many of the countries of the newer world. We continue to build urban hospitals for the fortunate minority and fail to provide finance for rural health centres to provide preventive medicine where it is needed for the less fortunate majority. In addition, the propensity of mankind to ignore any problem that is not obviously visible means that the 'unseen disability' of deafness, often more crippling than many more apparent handicaps, is relegated to second place.

None of us can deny that there is a major problem *What can we do?* In some wealthy countries of the developed world and in ideal circumstances the partially deaf are helped; a few by surgery, many by the consideration and care of both parents and teachers and some with hearing aids. The profoundly deaf attend schools for the deaf, probably the most expensive form of education in any country of the world and the only path for a deaf child to achieve his or her full potential.

The priorities for both these groups are early detection, early training and prevention of the disability. In many countries of the word, circumstances make these priorities, though no less valid, either impossible or too expensive to attain.

Hearing aids are simply not available to the great majority of deaf children in the world. The use of aids in most tropical countries is negligible. Hot, humid climates inactivate aids and destroy batteries with the speed, if not of light, at least of that of sound! In many countries the aids have to be kept at school so that when children return home for holidays or leave school for work the aids are left behind either for the use of other children or for safe keeping. Provision of a hearing aid often causes more disappointment than benefit as early failure and lack of local technical skill for repair or servicing means that the useful life of the aid is unbelievably short. Technicians trained in electronics and able to repair or service hearing aids are easily diverted by the larger profits to be earned in radio and television repair! Finally, in some poorer countries, thoughtful health authorities realise that the provision of hearing aids to a privileged few will lead to a demand that for financial reasons cannot be met and so rightly forbid the issue of even a limited number even when provided by voluntary donation. For a country spending more of its gross national product on health than, say, the United States, the logic of this sort of control is inescapable.

Reasonably early detection of deafness seems common in most countries of the world in both urban and rural communities. In Nigeria we found that 60% of profoundly deaf children attended for examination and opinion before 6 years of age and 24% before 2 years (table III). I believe that it is usual for deafness to be recognised by the mother or an elder sibling 'mother substitute' within the first year or so but the problems that the mother of a deaf child faces in most of the rural areas of the developing world are so intractable and overwhelming that the problems of an urban mother – not light by any means – are almost nothing in comparison. How does one manage to take a child from a

Table III. Age of deaf children referred to U.C.H. Ibadan

Age											Total
1	2	3	4	5	6–7	8–9	10–11	12–13	14–15	16+	
h											
13	47	38	31	21	34	21	22	14	7	5	253
% 5	19	15	12	8	13	8	9	6	3	2	

59% attend before 6 years of age.

Table IV. Ages of children seen at schools for the deaf and deaf units (where age was recorded)

		Age						Total
		6–7	8–9	10–11	12–13	14–15	16+	
All schools	n	86	79	91	96	49	39	440
	%	19.5	18	20.5	22	11	9	
Ilorin	n	6	8	14	20	16	13	77
	%	8	10	18	26	21	17	
All other schools	n	80	71	77	76	33	26	363
	%	22	20	21	21	9	7	

country village, perhaps a hundred miles to a clinic or hospital when the local transport runs once a week, or once a month if at all, and there is all the work of the family to do; trading, farming, cooking and probably another child at the breast? How does one manage a 2- or 3-day journey for a follow-up appointment? Weekly visits for parent and pre-school guidance can only be a dream. It is no wonder that perhaps only 2% of the deaf eventually reach a school for the deaf and the possibility of special education.

Special education at a school for the deaf, if, despite all difficulties a child should gain a place, is rarely started early enough. We found in Nigeria that only 20% of children in schools for the deaf were between 6 and 7 years of age in Ibadan, a large city. In a country district, Ilorin, no more than 6% of children were as young as this (table IV).

It appears, therefore, that the great majority of deaf children in the world have little opportunity of using a hearing aid. When on rare occasions an aid becomes available the chances of keeping it in working order or even of obtaining batteries are very small. Early recognition of deafness seems usual, but in only a tragically small number of cases is early diagnosis followed by early education – often commenced long after the child has become a 'fixed visualiser'.

Many otologists know these facts as well or better than I. It is unrealistic, I feel, to talk of the issue of hearing aids, early admission to special schools, peripatetic counselling for parents and pre-school guidance as if this is at all possible for the many at the present time or in the forseeable future as it is – in some wealthy countries – for the few.

All is not dark. I believe that we should concentrate our minds and effort on the third priority; the identification of the causes of deafness and the prevention of the disability. In 1981, Prof. *Victor Goodhill* wrote to me from California: 'Some major changes are evident in pediatric hearing losses here in Southern California. There is great reduction in paediatric sensorineural hearing loss. Our schools for the deaf are closing in many communities. Rubella, rhesus deafness, meningitis are all decreasing.'

California is surely one of the places in the world where preventive medicine has reached its highest level of technique. If as a result schools for the deaf are actually being closed down for lack of pupils, this must be a sign for the rest of the world. It is far cheaper and more cost-effective to prevent deafness than to build, staff and run these most expensive of all special schools.

Taking the causes of deafness in general it is probable that more than half the causative factors are potentially if not actually preventable. The exact proportions of the various factors will differ from continent to continent though all will play some part in every nation and community. It may be of interest to take some major preventable cause and relate each to a different continent, remembering that each though of special importance in that part of the world is by no means specific to that area.

Infective Disease and Africa

Infectious middle ear disease is, of course, common in many tropical countries but the degree of deafness is often minor or moderate and

Table V. Causes of deaths in childhood in West Africa

Cause	n	Cause	n
Malaria	76	enteric	27
Measles	51	meningococcus	7
TB	33	nonmeningitis	
Tetanus	33	meningitis	17

28% are due to infective disease (figures/1,000).

Table VI. Age of acquisition of deafness in measles and meningitis

Deafness		Age											Total
		infancy	1	2	3	4	5	6	7	8	9	10+	
All cause	n	55	59	41	27	20	16	12	7	4	2	11	254
	%	22	23	16	11	8	6	5	3	1.5	0.5	4	
Meningitis	n	8	13	8	9	4	5	3	2			8	60
	%	13	22	13	15	7	8	5	3			13	
Measles	n	31	27	17	7	4	6	3	1	2		1	99
	%[1]												

[1] % figures the same.

our efforts are largely directed to safety rather than to restoration of function. It is attractive to think of 'ear camps' to correspond with the 'eye camps' where cataract surgery and corneal grafting restores sight, but sadly the results of tympanoplasty do not warrant taking surgery to the rural area nor is the degree of deafness as a result of otitis media often really a serious handicap in a rural environment. The infectious diseases that cause profound sensorineural deafness are of much greater importance – in West Africa a third of the children die from infectious disease, malaria and measles coming high on the list (table V). Meningitis and enteric disease are also important killers and all these infections are reported to affect the inner ear. Almost two thirds of the deaf children in Ibadan, where it was possible to attribute a cause for the deafness, were deafened by measles, meningitis and rubella in

Table VII. Meningitis deafness in Africa (percentage of the total deaf)

Meningitis	Otitis media	Unknown	Author
22	14	37	*Couldrey*, 1968
16	15	30	*Clifford*, 1968
5	2	68	*Oyemade*, 1975
18	6	38	*Holborow*, 1979
24	8	30	*Holborow*, 1979

about equal proportions. As always, measles affects a very young population while meningitis occurs at a later age (table VI, VII).

Other infectious diseases – malaria, cytomegalovirus infection and enteric disease warrant much more thorough investigation with regard to inner ear damage. Malaria, the commonest killer of children, may simply potentiate the effect of other diseases or it may cause damage to the microvascular circulation of the inner ear. Cytomegalovirus acts, like the rubella virus, on the developing foetus and is thought by some to be even more important. Enteric disease is reported by *Kakar* [1975] to be of considerable importance in India. In a series of 210 cases, post-enteric deafness was found to be the second most frequent cause. It would of great interest to know more of this problem and further investigation and information is greatly to be hoped for.

Genetic Deafness and the Indian Subcontinent

Figures as high as 70% [*Kapur*, 1968] and 80% [*Kameswaran*, 1975] have been given as the percentage of children with genetically determined deafness at some schools in India. It is clear that genetic factors may influence susceptibility to both infections [*Anderson* et al., 1970] and to acoustic trauma but figures of this very high level are not found elsewhere. Consanguinous marriages are part of the culture and custom in many parts of the Indian subcontinent and Asia and, of course, also continue to be the custom in the expatriate communities in Africa. Genetic deafness is present in a larger proportion in East Africa where there are many Indian families, than in West Africa where marriages within the family do not take place.

The problems of genetically-determined deafness are among the most difficult in medicine; though it is theoretically possible to reduce disabilities in this field, parental counselling and an attempt to alter a people's way of life may not be readily accepted. In addition a considerable proportion of hereditary deafness is due to autosomal-recessive mechanisms so counselling can only be given after the birth of a deaf child.

Acoustic Trauma and the Industrial and Developed World

In the so-called developed world noise-induced permanent threshold shift of hearing is common in the industrial work force. Acoustic trauma is wholly untreatable and entirely preventable. It is estimated that there are 100,000 people in the United Kingdom with severe deafness from acoustic trauma and the United States is paying war veterans more in pensions for deafness than for any other disability.

Though noise-induced deafness is an increasing problem in industrial nations and communities it must not be thought that rural communities in agricultural countries are exempt. The Trinidad steel-band players show audiographs with a total cut-off above 2,000 cps, workers in sugar-crushing mills and those who beat out old oil drums for recycling in remote parts of the world are all subject to the same damage and disability.

What of the Future?

Deafness is such a crippling handicap and our efforts to help the deaf are so time consuming and expensive that prevention of deafness must always be more practical and more cost-effective than treatment. The more rural and underprivileged the community, the more this conclusion is forced upon us and I have tried to show that the great majority of the deaf in the world fall into this underprivileged category.

Immunisation, undertaken on a routine but intermittent basis, even with the constraints imposed by the 'cold chain', is often possible where other forms of medical care cannot be easily delivered. The deafness of acoustic trauma is a matter of continual health education while genetically induced deafness – infinitely more difficult to control – is also potentially preventable by continued education.

The responsibility for the education of governments towards preventive immunisation, individuals to protect their ears from noise and peoples to change (inevitably slowly) their way of life devolves on the otologist. He – or she – alone of all specialists knows best the effect of the 'unseen disability' of deafness, so often overlooked, on the development of the individual and he cannot, in all conscience, turn back to his microscope and the fascinating and important subject of otitis media without some thought to the wider problem.

The Expanded Programme on Immunisation of WHO, designed to control six infectious diseases by 1990, is of great importance – rubella immunisation has yet to be fully considered in this programme and I believe should have a place. The control of this disease and the other infectious deafness-producing diseases is a priority task.

May I conclude with two quotations: *Victor Goodhill:* 'Our schools for the deaf are closing in many communities', and *Robert Kennedy:* 'We all of us stand in the gutter. Some of us look at our feet and say "Why". Other look at the stars and say "Why Not"?'

References

Anderson, H.; Barr, B.; Wedenberg, E.: Genetic disposition – A prerequisite for maternal rubella deafness. Archs Otolar. *91:* 141 (1970).

Clifford, P.: Causes of deafness in Africa, p. 54. Report of Kenya Seminar on Deafness (Commonwealth Society for the Deaf, London 1968).

Couldrey, E.: Speech and hearing problems in Kenya, p. 58. Report of Kenya Seminar on Deafness (Commonwealth Society for the Deaf, London 1968).

Holborow, C.; Martinson, F.; Anger, N.: A study of deafness in West Africa (Commonwealth Society for the Deaf and Commonwealth Foundation, London 1981).

Holborow, C.: Problems of deafness in the developing countries. Proc. 4th Asia-Oceania Congr. Oto-Rhino-Laryngology (OLSA, Sydney 1979).

Kakar, P.K.: Sensori-neural deafness and its prevention; in Problems of deafness in the newer world. Proc. Semin. Commonw. Soc. for the Deaf, University of Sussex, p. 105 (Commonwealth Foundation, London 1975).

Kameswaran, S.: ENT diseases in a tropical environment, p. 129 (Higginbothams, Madras, 1975).

Kapur, Y.P.: Study of the aetiology and pattern of deafness in a school for the deaf in Madras, South India. Proc. Congr. Wld Fed. of Deaf, Warsaw 1967.

Oyemade, A.: The care of deaf schoolchildren and other handicapped in Nigeria. J. R. Soc. Hlth. *95:* 282 (1975).

Christopher Holborow, MD, ENT Department, Westminster Hospital, St. John's Gardens, London SW1 (UK)

Adv. Oto-Rhino-Laryng., vol. 29, pp. 183–193 (Karger, Basel 1983)

Methods of Early Identification of Hearing-Impaired Children

Gunnar Lidén, Aira Kankkunen

Departments of Audiology and Otolaryngology, Sahlgren's Hospital, University of Göteborg, Sweden

In order to identify and habilitate deaf and hard-of-hearing children as early as possible, a joint program has been in operation between pediatricians and the ENT and Audiology Department, Sahlgren's Hospital, Göteborg, since 1970. The program is composed of the following activities: (1) Identification of high-risk infants by pediatricians at the maternity hospitals. The babys are referred to us for hearing evaluation which is done at an age of 4 months. (2) All parents with a newborn baby receive a brochure about the normal child's hearing and language development [Audiology Department, 1970]. This may alert the parents to ask for medical advice if their child does not develop normally. (3) Well-baby clinics screen for hearing loss at an age of 7–9 months and again at an age of 4 years. (4) The pediatricians at the children's hospital refer all children after serious diseases as meningitis, sepsis, and after treatment with ototoxic drugs and whenever hearing loss is suspected. (5) Parents who suspect hearing loss or delayed language and speech development in their child can also come directly to the Audiology Department. (6) Referrals receive a hearing assessment in the Audiology Department.

The purpose of the present investigation is to report the results of our identification program during the last 10 years. This is done by analyzing the efficiency of the high-risk register in identifying children with impaired hearing in Göteborg compared to other sources, i.e. well-baby clinics and parents; the age of diagnosis; the initiators of the first hearing evaluation; the etiology; the frequency and degree of hearing impairment.

Table I. High-risk criteria used by maternity hospitals in Göteborg, 1970–1979

 1 Family history of hearing impairment
 2 Rubella or some other viral disease during the first half of pregnancy
 3 Multiple malformations particularly of the face and ears
 4 Immaturity (birth weight less than 2,500 g)
 5 Serum bilirubin more than 340 μmol/l (20 mg%) for newborns, not diagnosed as immature
 6 Serum bilirubin more than 255 μmol/l (15 mg%) for newborns with the diagnosis of immaturity
 7 Anoxia or neurological symptoms of cerebral origin for more than 24 h
 8 Congenital infections
 9 Diabetes mellitus in the mother
10 Hypoglycemia

Material

The pediatricians at the maternity hospitals in Göteborg have referred about 350 high-risk infants each year for hearing assessment. The high-risk criteria used by the maternity hospitals when we started the program 10 years ago (table I) [*Hirsch and Kankkunen*, 1974] conformed closely to the guidelines of the American Joint Committee on Newborn Hearing Screening [1972, 1974; *Davis, 1965; Mencher,* 1976; *Gerber,* 1977; *Gerber and Mencher,* 1978]. During a 10-year period (1970–1980) 3,531 high-risk children out of 57,172 born had their hearing assessed with respiration and observation audiometry [*Kankkunen and Lidén,* 1977, 1981]. 30 (0.8%) of the high-risk infants showed hearing loss of varying degree [*Kankkunen and Lidén,* 1982]. During the same period from 1970 to 1980, a total of 179 children were diagnosed as deaf or hard-of-hearing.

Methods

The risk babys are tested at an age of 4 months with tone and impedance audiometry. The tone audiogram is obtained by using a respiration and/or an observation audiometry technique [*Kankkunen and Lidén,* 1977]. Tympanometry and stapedius reflex test with ipsilateral stimulation are used for middle ear evaluation. In 1- to 2½-year-old children visual reinforcement audiometry [*Lidén and Kankkunen,* 1969] is the method of choice and in the age period 2½ to 6 years play audiometry [*Barr,* 1955] is commonly used.

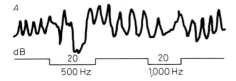

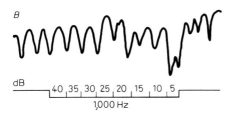

Fig. 1. The result of respiration audiometry of a 3-month-old infant. *A* The breathing pattern changes clearly upon stimulation with faint tones. *B* Stimulation with tones of decreasing intensity. The changes in the breathing are clearest at low levels [from *Kankkunen and Lidén,* 1977].

Respiraton audiometry provides an accurate determination of the tone threshold in children during the neonatal and early infancy ages. The method requires little preparation of the child and is therefore well suited for outpatient practice. In order for the test to be reliable it must be carried out in a soundproof room. Upon the introduction of acoustic stimulation, the breathing pattern of the child becomes irregular, shallower or deeper. Since 1971 we have been using impedance-plethysmography in order to record changes in breathing rhythm due to acoustic stimulation. Sudden acoustic stimuli will make the baby 'catch his breath'. If the child is listening to a faint sound, arrested breathing eliminates disturbing respiratory sounds. For the recording of the child's breathing rhythm an electrode is placed on both sides of the child's chest and fed with weak high-frequency (100 kHz) current. The breathing movements change the air volume of the lungs and, in doing so, also change the impedance. Such changes in impedance can be recorded as voltage variation reflecting the breathing rhythm. The voltage variations between the electrodes are amplified and recorded by a recorder. A typical result of respiration audiometry on a 3-month-old infant is shown in figure 1. Respiration audiometry makes it possible in about 90% to ascertain an infant's hearing. The reliability is good as is demonstrated in figure 2.

Visual reinforcement audiometry is presumably well known as it is a modification of the conditioned orientation reflex audiometry by *Suzuki and Ogiba* [1961].

Age of Diagnosis: the number of children diagnosed annually as well as their age at the first investigation are listed in table II. As can be seen, only 52% of the hearing-impaired children were diagnosed at an age of 2 years.

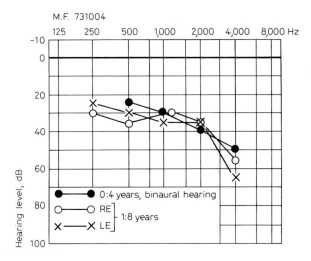

Fig. 2. The results of respiration audiometry on a 4-month-old infant. Sound stimulation via loudspeaker. Binaural hearing. Visual reinforcement audiometry on same child at an age of 1 year 8 months [from *Kankkunen and Lidén*, 1977].

Initiators for the First Hearing Evaluation

Considering our relatively well-established health and welfare system, it was of interest to identify the initiators of the first hearing evaluation. As can be seen in table III, only 17% were high-risk children from the maternity hospitals, 28% came from well-baby clinics, 24% from children's hospitals and other medical centers. To our surprise the largest referral group came directly from the parents (31%).

Etiology

To shed light of the efficiency of the high-risk criteria in detecting hearing-handicapped children, the cause of deafness and hearing impairment was analyzed both in the high-risk group as well as in the total group of 179 children. The cause of hearing impairment among the 30 children referred as high-risk infants are shown in table IV. As can be seen, the risk factors were obvious in 28 (93%) of 30 infants as deaf parents, malformed ears, rubella matris and meningitis. 2 of the high-risk infants had neonatal disease. One of them was small-for-date, had

Table II. 179 children identified as deaf or hard of hearing in Göteborg (1970–1980) in relation to age at diagnosis

Age at diagnosis	n	%
0–0:11	65	36
1–1:11	29	16
2–2:11	18	10
3–3:11	14	8
4–4:11	25	14
5–5:11	22	13
6–6:11	6	3
Total	179	100

Table III. Initiators of the first hearing evaluation

	n	%
Maternity hospitals	30	17
Well-baby clinic	50	28
Children's hospital	26	15
Otolaryngologists	8	4
Speech pathologists	9	5
Parents	56	31
Total	179	100

cerebral anoxia postpartum and hypoglycemia. The second one had hyperbilirubinemia (278 μmol/l), and a birth weight of 1,150 g. In both families heredity was a factor in the hearing impairment. Genetic factors could be established in 17 (57%) of the 30 children.

Genetic factors are also dominant in the total group of 179 hearing-impaired children (table V). Heredity appeared to be the only cause of hearing impairment in 42%, and when combined with other causes it was present in an additional 12%. Stated differently, genetic factors were present in 54% of all the hearing-impaired children. Nonhereditary causes amounted to 29% of our group. These children and those combining heredity with other causes were suffering from hearing loss

Table IV. Etiology of hearing impairment in 30 children referred as high-risk infants

Year of birth	Deaf parent	Malformed ear	Rubella matris	Neonatal disease	Meningitis	Total
1970	–	3	1 (+)	–	–	4
1971	2	2 (+)	–	–	–	4
1972	–	1	–	1 (+)	–	2
1973	–	2	1 (+)	1 (+)	–	4
1974	1	–	–	–	–	1
1975	1	–	–	–	–	1
1976	4	1	–	–	–	5
1977	–	–	–	–	–	–
1978	2	2	–	–	1	5
1979	1	2	1	–	–	4
Total	11	13	3	2	1	30

(+) = Heredity for hearing loss.

Table V. Causes of hearing impairment in 179 hearing-impaired children

	n		%
Heredity	74	} 97	54
Heredity and other causes	23		
Other causes	52		29
Unknown	30		17
Total	179		100

due to ear malformations, meningitis, parotitis and rubella matris. Only 7 (4%) children of the 179 had a history of neonatal disease. 3 children had meningitis or sepsis, 2 had cerebral anoxia and 2 had hyperbilirubinemia due to Rh- and ABO-hemolytic disease. Only 1 of the children suffering from anoxia had 65 dB hearing loss. The other 6 children had only mild sensorineural high frequency loss.

30 children were classified as having hearing impairment of unknown origin. Most of them were very young. As deafness is a serious handicap it is not uncommon that questioning parents about genetic

Table VI. Degree and frequency of hearing losses in 115 6-year-old children born 1970–1974 in relation to 31,280 live births in Göteborg during same period

Hearing loss, dB	Children, n	%	‰ of 31,280 births
< 25 (0.5–2.0 kHz)	4	3	0.1
25–40	41	36	1.3
41–60	16	14	0.5
61–100	15	13	0.5
> 100	5	4	0.2
Deafness	2	2	0.1
Monaural hearing loss	9	8	0.3
Monaural deafness	23	20	0.7
Total	115	100	3.7

factors yield negative responses because of guilt and anxiety. Gradually the parent may come to accept their child's hearing handicap and thus hereditary factors can be more easily revealed. Audiometric identification of normal-hearing carriers of genes of deafness according to *Anderson and Wedenberg* [1968] is also offered to most of the parents. Further, it can be mentioned that 5 children in this group were adopted from foreign countries.

Frequency and Degree of Hearing Impairment

The frequency and degree of hearing loss vary among the children partly depending on the age of diagnosis. The number of children identified as hearing impaired at a certain age unfortunately does not always coincide with the prevalence of hearing impairment in the age population. For many reasons it was of interest to determine the frequency and degree of hearing loss in 6-year-old children. In our material of 179 hearing-impaired children born 1970–1980, 115 6-year-olds (born 1970–1974) have been analyzed in relation to the total number of 31,280 live births in Göteborg in the same period (table VI). The frequency of hearing impairment amounted to 3.7‰. The investigation showed also that 0.3‰ were ranked as deaf, 1.3‰ had a hearing loss worse than 40 dB HL, 2.4‰ had a mild hearing loss, i.e. less than

Table VII. Degree and frequency of hearing losses in 64 children born 1975–1979 in relation to 25,892 live births in Göteborg during same period in December 1980

Hearing loss, dB	Children, n	%	‰ of 25,892 births
< 25 (0.5–2.0 kHz)	3	5	0.1
25–40	23	36	0.9
41–60	5	8	0.2
61–100	7	11	0.3
> 100	3	5	0.1
Deafness	6	9	0.2
Monaural hearing loss	11	17	0.4
Monaural deafness	6	9	0.2
Total	64	100	2.5

40 dB HL in the best ear, or monaural hearing loss or monaural deafness. The majority of the children had hearing loss of genetic origin. This type of hearing loss has a tendency to get worse, which means that some of them with mild to moderate losses will move down in the table.

The remaining group of 64 hearing-impaired children born during 1975–1979 have different ages from 1 to 5 years. The degree of their hearing impairment as established in December 1980 is shown in table VII. The frequency of hearing impairment in this group related to the total number of 25,892 live births during the same period amounts to 2.5‰. Hearing loss worse than 60 dB HL is found in 0.6‰. Comparing these figures with those from the 6-year-olds (born 1970–1974) which amounted to 3.7 and 0.8‰, respectively, we can expect that the present number of hearing-impaired children will rise when these age groups have reached an age of 6 years.

Discussion

When we started our high-risk program as a substitute for mass newborn hearing testing we hoped to increase identification sensitivity. On the basis of our 10-year survey we feel, however, disappointed [*Kankkunen and Lidén,* 1981]. 6% of all newborns failed the risk criteria and were judged at risk to develop hearing loss. Our investigation,

Table VIII. Criteria for hearing control

Prenatal
Heredity for hearing loss
Rubella and other viral infections during first half of pregnancy
Malformation of ears and/or face
Chromosome aberrations
Unclear syndromes

Perinatal
Birth weight less than 1,500 g
Serious asphyxia requiring at least 10 min resuscitation and all respirator-treated children
Neonatal sepsis/meningitis

Postnatal
Meningitis
Parotitis

---

however, showed that only 30, i.e. 0.8% of the risk children had a hearing loss of varying degree. Only 30 (17%) of the 179 hearing-impaired children came through the high-risk register. 28 of 30 infants were obviously at risk to develop or show hearing loss: that is, deaf parents, malformation of ears or face, rubella matris or meningitis. These children would probably have been identified and diagnosed even without the high-risk register. Asphyxia and hyperbilirubinemia are associated with only a mild hearing loss, or none at all. As a result of our experiences we have revised the high-risk criteria and now recommend hearing control according to table VIII.

In this new criterion hyperbilirubinemia, diabetes mellitus in the mother and hypoglycemia have been excluded. Children with serious asphyxia requiring of least 10 min resuscitation and all respirator-treated children as well as those with immaturity and a birth weight less than 1,500 g are still considered at risk. However, it should be mentioned that during an 8-year period, 137 children with a birth weight less than 1,500 g have survived. Of these only 4 had a mild hearing loss of about 30 dB HL. Even if the high-risk register has not been very efficient up to now, we feel that we cannot do without it, especially if we use the revised form. We feel this revised form will strengthen the sensitivity of the high-risk register.

The analysis of the material also showed that most of the children

Table IX. Memento to the staff of well-baby clinics concerning hearing loss in children

---

Take an elaborate anamnesis concerning hearing loss among the child's relatives
Watch regularly for the child's reactions on sound and voice
Use a selective attention test with calibrated sound sources at an age of 7–9 months and
    at about 2 years of age
Use tone screening at the compulsory 4-years health control
Observe continuously the child's hearing and language development
Listen to the mother's suspicion of her child having communicative problems
Refer all children with suspicion of hearing loss immediately for hearing assessment

---

(31%) had their hearing loss identified through the parents and only 28% through well-baby clinics and 24% from other medical centers. This is astonishing in view of the present situation in Göteborg where the well-baby clinics regularly check 94% of all children from birth up to 6 years of age. In order to improve the staff's ability of early identification of communicative disorders they are constantly encouraged to follow the protocol outlined in table IX. We have, among other things, found it important to provide the staff with a simple method for observing the child's reaction to sound. A calibrated 3,000-Hz warble tone instrument as well as the selective attention test BOEL [*Stensland Junker*, 1972] are very useful and should regularly be used not only at an age of 7–9 months but again at about 2 years of age. At the compulsory health control at an age of 4 years tone screening should be used. With a well-trained staff at the well-baby clinics an unnecessary delay in referral of children with impaired hearing will hopefully be rare.

Conclusions

Many risk factors in the existing high-risk criteria have been shown to be unneeded and are excluded in the revised form which is presented. To avoid unnecessary delay in the referral of children with impaired hearing a close cooperation with the pediatrician is necessary. The well-baby clinics are encouraged to test the hearing of children regularly at an age of 7–9 months, and at about 2 and 4 years of age. Respiration audiometry is a reliable audiometric method in young infants. In small children visual reinforcement audiometry is the method of choice.

References

Anderson, H.; Wedenberg, E.: Audiometric identification of normal hearing carriers of genes of deafness. Acta oto-lar. *65:* 535 (1968).

Audiology Department, Sahlgren's Hospital and Children Health Care, Göteborg 1970: The ear, an important sense organ (in Swedish).

Barr, B.: Pure tone audiometry for preschool children. Acta otolar. suppl. 121 (1955).

Davis, H.: The young deaf child: identification and management. Acta otolar. suppl. 203 (1965).

Gerber, S.E.: High-risk registry for congenital deafness; in Jaffe, Hearing loss in children, pp. 74–77 (University Park Press, Baltimore 1977).

Gerber, S.; Mencher, G.: Early diagnosis of hearing loss (Grune & Stratton, New York 1978).

Hirsch, A.; Kankkunen, A.: High-risk history in the identification of hearing loss in newborns. Scand. Audiol. *3:* 177 (1974).

Joint Committee on Infant Hearing: Statement Asha *13:* 79 (1972).

Joint Committee on Infant Hearing: Supplementary statement Asha *16:* 160 (1974).

Kankkunen, A.; Lidén, G.: Respiration audiometry. Scand. Audiol. *6:* 81 (1977).

Kankkunen, A.; Lidén, G.: Wie effektiv ist das High-Risk-Register in der Früherkennung schwerhöriger Kinder? Sprache, Stimme, Gehör *5:* 39 (1981).

Kankkunen, A.; Lidén, G.: Early identification of hearing handicapped children. Acta otolar. suppl. 386, p. 31 (1982).

Lidén, G.; Kankkunen, A.: Visual reinforcement audiometry, Acta otolar. *67:* 281 (1969).

Mencher, G.: Early identification of hearing loss (Karger, Basel 1976).

Stensland Junker, K.: Selective attention in infants and consecutive communicative behavior (Almqvist & Wiksell, Stockholm 1972).

Suzuki, T.; Ogiba, Y.: Conditioned orientation reflex audiometry. Archs Otolar. *74:* 192 (1961).

G. Lidén, MD, Departments of Audiology and Otolaryngology,
Sahlgren's Hospital, University of Göteborg, S-41345 Göteborg (Sweden)

Adv. Oto-Rhino-Laryng., vol. 29, pp. 194–198 (Karger, Basel 1983)

Various Approaches for the Improvement of Hearing

Jun-Ichi Suzuki

Department of Otolaryngology, Teikyo University School of Medicine, Tokyo, Japan

Difficulties with speech and hearing are 'invisible disorders', which have difficult access and, therefore, are difficult to assess. Four approaches to the alleviation of such difficulties are discussed, namely, one method of examination or diagnosis of deafness and three different kinds of treatment, otomicrosurgery, hearing aids and middle ear implant.

Diagnostic difficulties in young children is the first problem. Speech therapists may help us in examining hearing in children. For examining deafness in young children using a behavioral hearing test, different kinds of toys that create noise are utilized. It should be noted that the respective frequencies of these sounds vary widely. Thus, objective methods, in addition to these subjective ones, are indispensable.

Among recently developed methods for such objective assessment, the auditory brain stem response (ABR) has proved to be most useful and reliable and, as such, essential (fig. 1). In addition to the advantages already mentioned, the ABR, when present, is easily detectable even by non-specialists. The thresholds with different frequencies, such as 500, 1,000, 2,000 and 4,000 Hz, can be determined by the ABR and, as anticipated, are actually close to those determined behaviorally.

In infants less than 12 months of age, however, the situation is different. While the ABR test can be applied to children of any age, the behavioral tests, especially a reliable one, cannot. Thus, there may be some discrepancy between the thresholds obtained by the ABR and those by behavioral audiometry, and this has to be explained in each case. Children with suspected deafness will come to the clinic and sit for various auditory examinations. In our university hospital so far,

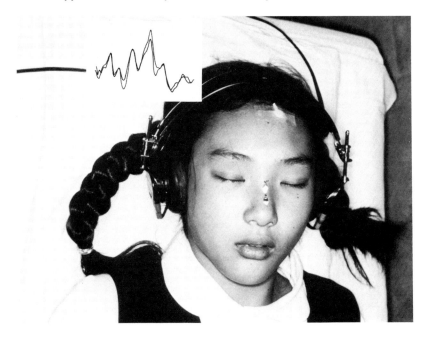

Fig. 1. ABR being recorded during a child's sleep.

the majority of such children have been 1 year old. Apart from the ABR, auditory evoked responses with different latencies in general appear to be useful for analyzing pathophysiological processes at different levels along the auditory pathways in the CNS. This is an area of research that I believe will be very promising to explore.

Speech processes in the cerebral cortex and their close relationship with hearing are now a target of research for otolaryngologists and are more important than ever before. Thus, more sophisticated experimental psychological approaches are needed, and are becoming available.

After more than 20 years of trial and error, otomicrosurgery has become very dependable as a technique for the improvement of conductive deafness. In general, chronic otitis media with a central perforation is the easiest subject for otomicrosurgery. Namely, otorrhea can be alleviated without difficulty in almost every case and, in most, hearing also can be improved.

Among other conditions, microtia is an important and still challenging target for otologists. In this connection, we were struck by a

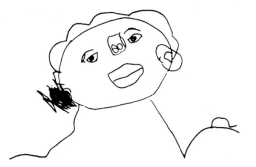

Fig. 2. A drawing by a 5-year-old girl with microtia.

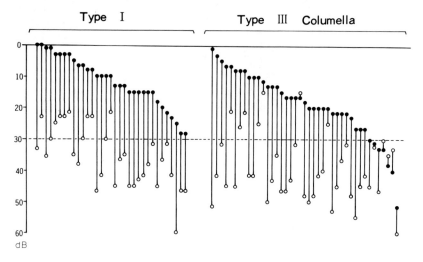

Fig. 3. Average hearing thresholds before (○) and after (●) type I and type III Columella tympanoplasties.

drawing by a 5-year-old child with microtia, indicating the youngster's severe preoccupation with her abnormal ear (fig. 2).

Frequently, middle ear effusion in children is not an easy disorder to control, starting with difficulty in detection and ending with the effects of this condition on the child's intellectual and emotional development. Furthermore, adhesive otitis media and extensive middle ear sclerosis can result from middle ear effusion. This is probably also true for attic cholesteatoma. Both tympanosclerosis and cholesteatoma may completely destroy middle ear functions. The average air- and

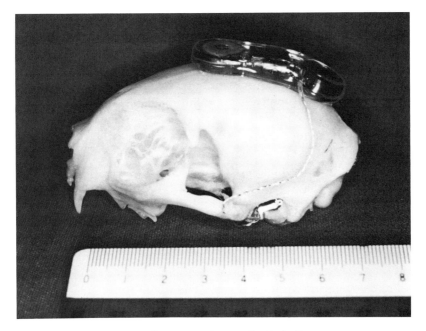

Fig. 4. A middle ear implant for a cat on the top of cat's skull.

bone-conduction thresholds in chronic otitis media are 50 and 10 dB, respectively. Tympanoplasty, which has become increasingly successful and safe, should be applied to chronic otitis media.

Let me compare two types of tympanoplasty, type I and type III with columella, both of which are common in our department. Figure 3 shows the average recovery course of hearing after these two types of tympanoplasty. These recovery courses appeared to be parallel, but there were distinct differences between them. Statistics also showed that the postoperative threshold was usually less than 30 dB and slightly lower in type I than in type III.

In discussing hearing aids, it should be noted that those most commonly used by adults, and this is probably true in any country of the world, are the behind-the-ear type. The hearing aid clinic in our hospital has been very busy since it was opened 5 years ago: both patients and hearing aids have to be repeatedly examined and assessed, and the patients have to be continuously encouraged and monitored. Therefore, efforts related to fitting of hearing aids have come to be highly evaluated. Recently, for example, about 50% of the patients' old hearing aids have become applicable by going through the hearing aid clinic.

I will now give a brief report on the Japanese government project aimed at implanting hearing aids. Since recently developed hearing aids have become increasingly miniaturized while still being very effective, it is natural to consider implanting them in the ear in order to avoid the many inconveniences associated with their use. This concept is rapidly becoming a reality in Japan and, hopefully, can be applied in the near future. In this connection, a microphone, an amplifier, a battery and a vibrator (attached to the stapes head) will all be implanted. It was fortunate that a ceramic vibrator was found to have both sufficient power for this purpose as well as high-fidelity frequency response.

Early in 1981, a model for a cat was completed, and the middle-ear implant undertaken 6 months ago is still functioning well. The cat model has a microphone-amplifier-battery complex and is implanted on the top of the skull (fig. 4). We anticipate that a model for humans will be developed within this year. The site of implantation of the battery-amplifier complex in humans will be the temporal muscle area.

Since the project was started 4 years ago, we have successfully overcome many technical difficulties. In this connection, the ABR was one of the most important techniques in the evaluation of the implant. This is a 4½-year project of the Japanese government, and two companies, Rion Co., Ltd. and Sanyo Co., Ltd., are participating. A group of both medical and technological specialists has been assisting these firms. 1982 will be devoted to the final work on the technology-biology interphase, namely, on the actual implantation.

Jun-Ichi Suzuki, MD, Department of Otolaryngology,
Teikyo University School of Medicine, Kaga 2-11-1, Itabashi-ku, Tokyo (Japan)

Adv. Oto-Rhino-Laryng., vol. 29, pp. 199–208 (Karger, Basel 1983)

Early Fitting of Hearing Aids and Early Education for the Severely to Profoundly Hearing-Impaired Children

Hideo Imai

The National Institute of Special Education, Yokosuka, Kanagawa, Japan

As an educator, and not physician, for hearing-impaired patients, I believe it is necessary in this interdisciplinary field, that the physician, psychologist, social worker and educator or therapist are mutually cooperative for attaining good results. Some recent results involving the early education of hearing-impaired children are presented and it is hoped that they will deepen the mutual understanding between doctors and educators.

Fitting of the Hearing Aid

The first task of the school or clinic for hearing-impaired children is the fitting of hearing aids. Various kinds of hearing aids are in use throughout the world, e.g. body aid, behind-ear type aid, in-the-ear type aid or a hearing aid for babies, which I have modified from the behind-ear type aid. The performance of hearing aids is shown in figure 1, and includes frequency response, acoustic gain, maximum power output, distortion of the output, and if necessary, AGC characteristics.

Frequency responses are, roughly speaking, the measure to select the hearing aid corresponding to the type of audiogram, and the acoustic gain and maximum power output correspond to the value of the hearing level. When the hearing aid is fitted to the infant there are some problems which have to be considered, namely that (1) it is difficult to get other audiological data beyond the hearing thresholds; (2) the values of hearing thresholds are not definite, and (3) hearing aids are not manufactured suitably enough for children in the way of size, weight, etc.

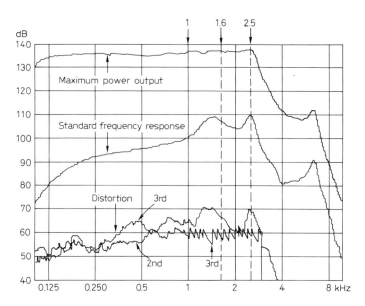

Fig. 1. Frequency response curves of a hearing aid.

Various considerations have to be made when fitting hearing aids to the infant; however, generally speaking, the hearing aid selected first is often tentative. At first I select wide-band type hearing aids with a flat gain or a slightly high-emphasized gain, the acoustic gain being about half of the hearing level, and the MPO of the aid being at the level of 120–130 dB SPL. Setting of the MPO at the correct (not-to-high) level is important to prevent further hearing deprivation due to the high output. It is usually necessary to readjust the characteristics of the fitted hearing aid, depending on the results of the tests that follow and of the mother's records of the observation of her child's auditory behavior in everyday life. Therefore, it is desirable that the hearing aid selected will be flexible in the term of changing the characteristics. From this point of view I would make use of the body-type hearing aid, even for the 1- to 2-year-old infant. We can adjust the frequency responses of a body-type hearing aid, controlling, for example, the tone circuit or replacing the earphone.

An example of the progress of fitting a hearing aid is given in table I. The child was 1½ years old when he first visited the clinic. The

Table I. The progress of fitting a hearing aid

Age: 1:6	age: 1:9		age: 1:11	age: 2:1
COR aud., dB	COR aud., dB		right ear:	with hearing aid
125 Hz: 40–50	250 Hz: 60–70		acoustic feedback	1 kHz: 75 dB
250 Hz: 75	500 Hz: 80		left ear:	cow bell: +
500 Hz: 90	1 kHz: 90 ╱		took off earphone	siren: +
Drum: +	2 kHz: 90 ╱		with loud voice	
Cow bell: ±	with hearing aid			
Siren: −	1 kHz: 75			
	loud voice: −			
Medium-power type hearing aid with semi-wide type earphone (vol. 4)	earphone: to peak-type	high-power type hearing aid with peak-type earphone	earphone: to wide-type	

hearing test results at admission are displayed on the left side of the table. At 125 Hz the hearing level was about 40–50 dB and at higher frequencies the levels were not certain. It seemed it was also true in the behavioral responses. A medium-powered hearing aid of flat gain was fitted, which is useful in utilizing low frequency information at first. After 3 months the hearing level showed 80 dB at 500 Hz. At higher frequencies it was not yet clear, so the earphone was replaced with a peaked-type one which emphasized the high frequency region. I tried to train and check the auditory behavior in this region with this hearing aid and also tried to change the hearing aid to a high-powered one with a peak-typed earphone. The results, however, were not positive. This hearing aid often caused acoustic feedback and the child took the earphone off when loud sounds were presented. The earphone was then changed to a wide-band response. The child was able to respond to some sounds in the high frequency region through the hearing aid.

Early Education

In Japan, there are 107 schools for the deaf and most of them have a nursery department for children from 3 years of age onwards and an

early guidance clinic for those under 3 years of age. At the nursery department, the teaching curriculum is composed following the general
curriculum of regular nursery schools, whereby the teaching of the language is emphasized. The children finishing the nursery department
enter the primary department or a regular school according to their
language ability and intelligence. As a general tendency, the severely or
profoundly handicapped children enter the primary department.

There are problems in the schools for the deaf in Japan. Pupils are,
generally speaking, much more delayed in language ability, so there is
also a delay in achievements in regular school subjects. The teachers
sometimes say that in this situation there is a barrier at the age of 9
which is difficult to get over. The causes of this delay are considered in
various ways. Early education from 3 years on started many years ago.
However, the results of the delay still remain. Of course, the earlier the
education begins, the better. However, is it alright when education
starts from under the age of 1 year? Is the oral method unsatisfactory in
conveying the information of language? Is the school system or the
curriculum not fitted to the education of the hearing-impaired children? What is the teacher competency nowadays?

Maximum Use of Hearing

For the language media, the general tendency in the world is towards total communication. Total communication utilizes all of the
language media, that is, hearing, lip-reading, gesture, fingerspelling
and sign language. The amount of information of language conveyed
with this method is much more than that with the oral method. We are
also researching the information content conveyed with the various
language media; hearing, lip-reading, cued speech and fingerspelling.
It has been confirmed that the fingerspelling method transmits the
maximum amount of information without any confusion. However,
on the other hand, it is said that the total communication is a 'philoso-
phy', and not 'total'. Especially auditory information is sometimes inhibited. From the audiological standpoint, we should try to utilize the
residual hearing as much as possible, because the auditory channel is
intrinsically related to the perception of speech, and also now, the
hearing aid can be fitted even to the severely and profoundly hearing-
impaired child.

Auditory Training

Many books have been written on the subject of auditory training. The sequence of the training usually follows the normal development of auditory function. The content is: awareness of sounds; localizing sounds; discriminating sounds; recognizing sounds; comprehending sounds; selecting a sound from background sounds, and auditory feedback to speech production.

At the earlier stages, the children freshly fitted with a hearing aid cannot attend and respond to sound well. The teacher has to teach them that there are sounds in the world and how to respond to said sounds. The functions of discriminating, recognizing and comprehending sounds are the most important functions for daily life activity. At first, training is usually performed by responding to a sound selected from a small set of stimuli, then to a large set and finally to an open set. The comprehension of the meaning of the stimuli and the children's response appropriate to its meaning in the daily life situation is the essential part of this step. Auditory feedback is also another essential feature of the auditory function. At first this function is formed from the imitation of the teacher's or mother's speech.

Utilization of Home Situation: Parent Education

Young children are taken care of and are brought up at home by their mothers. They learn daily life activity, their 'mother-tongue' and social behavior from the family. This home environment seems even more important for the hearing-impaired child, since learning in language which is one of the essential parts of the education of the hearing-impaired, will be accomplished through the real experiences repeated over and over again in real situations. It is supposed that this condition will not be satisfied in the school but in the home situation. However, it is absolutely indispensable to consider the special requirements of the hearing-impaired in the home situation, that is, to encourage every listening experience appropriate to the infant's hearing condition and every opportunity to utilize lip-reading or other means. These requirements come from the real fact that they have difficulties to hear even through the hearing aid and that they have to rely on other means for communication at the same time. Therefore, it will be essential to have the parent develop the ability to treat their infants at home; that is, parent education: teaching them and giving them practice of how to treat their children at home.

The program of parent education is called PIP (parent-infant program) in the USA. There are many PIPs in the United States, e.g. the PIP at CID in St. Louis, at the Bill-Wilkerson Hearing and Speech Center in Nashville. They all have the demonstration home which is a facility having the same functions as a regular home, that is, a dining kitchen, sitting room, bathroom, etc. Each mother-child pair visits the demonstration home once or twice a week and performs daily-life activities while being given instructions by the teacher.

At our Institute we also have a demonstration home and utilize it for our PIP. The activity is videorecorded and afterwards the teacher and the mother discuss the day's performance by watching the video.

Auditory Training at Home

As mentioned earlier, the utilization of the residual hearing is an essential part in the education of hearing-impaired children; however, sometimes it becomes a superficial one for the infant in the school situation. The following method is recommended in the home situation: (1) To utilize every opportunity and situation to teach the child the 'meaning' of the sound corresponding to the real situation in the flow of everyday life. For example, when the door bell rings by chance, the mother attracts the child's attention to the sound and waits for the bell to ring again, then welcomes the guest at the entrance. Thus, the child realizes the meaning of the bell ringing which is the signal that a guest visits his home and is welcomed by him. (2) To make use of a sound which is specially defined as the signal of a definite act. For example, a definite piece of music just before lunch starts. (3) Sound games, musical games, speech games guided pleasantly by the mother. These activites are programmed according to the child's achievement.

Results of the Parent-Infant Program in Japan

The National Institute of Special Education has been researching the Parent-Infant Program with the cooperation of the Mother-Child

Table II.

Age years: months at which they start their education	Mean hearing loss of better ear, dB (ISO)					Total
	70–79	80–89	90–99	100–109	110–119	
0:0–0:11				1		1
1:0–1:11		2	5	9	1	17
2:0–2:11	1	2		1	1	5
3:0–3:11		1				1
Total	1	5	5	11	2	24

Table III.

Age (years:months) after the hearing aid was fitted	Reacting to sounds
0:0–0:2	turning face to the source of loud sounds; watching the mother's face when she speaks
0:2–0:10	looking around searching for the source of sound
0:6–1:2	reacting to the sounds from outdoors
0:8–1:8	becoming sensitive to soft sounds
1:2–2:2	having a listening attitude and becoming sensitive to environmental sounds
1:2–2:0	responding to unfamiliar sounds by inquiring

Clinic for the Hearing Impaired. The number of children we have treated is 24 (table II). They are on the level above 70 dB in hearing and most of them started their education from 1 year of age onwards. They were given group training and parent practice at the Mother-Child Clinic once a week, and some of them attended the demonstration home at the Institute once every 2 weeks.

We followed their development in the reception of sounds and speech and the development of expressive language from the mothers' records of their children's development. Tables III–V show the receptive development of the severely and profoundly handicapped children according to the months after the hearing aids were fitted. After they develop the ability to attend to sound, they gradually recognize the sounds familiar in daily life, for example a door bell, a telephone bell

Table IV.

Age, years:months	Recognizing sounds
0:4–2:0	recognizing the doorbell and going to the entrance
0:7–3:0	recognizing the telephone ringing and making it known to the mother
0:8–1:2	discriminating between sounds of some musical instruments
1:0–1:9	discriminating between the cries of animals
3:5–3:11	recognizing most of the sounds familiar to him in daily life

Table V.

Age, years:months	Recognizing speech
0:2–0:9	understanding 'give me', 'bye bye'
0:3–1:5	understanding 'bow wow', 'beep beep', etc.
0:4–0:6	understanding the word for inhibition
0:11–1:8	understanding 'mama' or other family names
1:0–2:5	understanding his own name
1:9–2:8	understanding simple words or sentences in daily life
2:7–3:2	being interested in listening to the telephone and understanding simple sentences

ringing. They also develop the ability to recognize speech, from the words familiar to infants; 'give me', 'bye bye', and their name, greetings, familiar words in daily life and afterwards sentences. Their auditory memory of sounds and speech increased gradually. We have designed a new test to check the children's receptive ability to environmental sounds. In test I the child points to the things in the picture corresponding to the sounds heard. In test II the child points to the stimulus sound from a group of six pictures.

The vertical axis of figure 2 represents the correct scores and the horizontal axis represents the mean hearing level. Generally speaking these results show a higher correct score for our children than the other children. Also the hearing ability of our children when using a word list at the age of 5–6 is shown in figure 3. Some superiority of our children may be seen against the children attending the school for the deaf. These results verify the effects of the early utilization of residual hear-

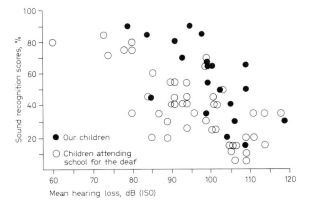

Fig. 2. Sound recognition ability of our children.

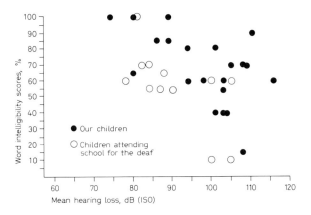

Fig. 3. Word recognition ability of our children.

ing and the early education emphasized in home training. In other words, the children attending the schools for the deaf have the potentiallity to recognize more sounds and speech.

Speech development is shown in tables VI and VII. Speech behavior starts from voicing under the auditory feedback through the hearing aid, then progresses to the stage of imitation then to the stage of spontaneous speech from individual words to the stage of complex sentences. We have also checked their receptive and expressive language ability with a standardized checklist. For example, item No. 1 of the list is 'Being startled with loud sounds or sudden sounds'. Item No. 10,

Table VI.

Age, years:months	Vocalizing and imitating
0:0–0:4	vocalizing naturally
0:2–1:5	vocalizing with inflecting intonation or various loudnesses
0:3–1:3	vocalizing to show his will, etc.
0:4–1:4	beginning jargon
0:2–1:5	imitating rhythm and intonation
0:5–1:1	imitating simple words

Table VII.

Age, years:months	Spontaneous speech
0:3–0:7	saying 'bye bye' and waving hand
0:5–0:8	saying 'mama'
0:3–0:11	saying 'bow wow', etc.
0:10–1:9	responding to calling his name and saying 'yes'
0:9–1:9	answering simple questions with one word
1:0–2:5	using two-word sentences and then multi-word sentences

which corresponds to 10 months after birth, is 'When he is asked where is beep-beep or where is mama?, he turns his face to the object'.

We can recognize their delay in language reception from a chart. However, though the appearance of each passing age is of course different in the individual, roughly speaking, the developmental stage in the cecklist has appeared after the start of education and the tendency shows their approaching normal development.

Conclusion

The utilization of residual hearing together with early education which has emphasis on the parent education have proved to be effective even with severely and profoundly hearing-impaired children.

H. Imai, MD, The National Institute of Special Education,
2360, Nobi, Yokosuka, Kanagawa-ken 239 (Japan)

Adv. Oto-Rhino-Laryng., vol. 29, pp. 209–215 (Karger, Basel 1983)

Speech Rehabilitation in Japan

Taiko Nagasawa

The National Institute of Special Education, Yokosuka, Kanagawa, Japan

I am a speech pathologist who has been working with the speech handicapped for about 20 years, both in the field of medicine and in the field of education. When I started working in this field, there were only a few people who were interested in speech disorders, although the needs were no less than today.

In the field of education, special help to speech-handicapped children had long been given by considerate classroom teachers after their classes were over. But it was not until 1958 that the first special speech class was established in the Japanese public school system. During the next decades, the number of special classes increased slowly. In the late 1950s and early 1960s, many parents of speech-handicapped children moved to the area where the child could have speech therapy. Since most fathers remained at their original residences in order to maintain their occupations, mothers and their handicapped children were forced to live separately.

The parents founded an association and they ardently and strongly requested the Ministry of Education and the local government to open speech classes in local schools. This parents' association was the moving force in convincing the government to establish speech classes all over Japan. The number rapidly increased in the 1970s. At present, there are more than 1,300 classes in about 1,000 schools. About 2,000 teachers are treating more than 20,000 children.

In 1968, the first 4-year course in a university was founded to train special speech teachers. At present, four universities have 4-year courses and two provide graduate programs, and eight universities have 1-year courses for in-service training.

A procedure for speech therapy in schools, taking articulation disorders as an example, is as follows. When we first meet children with articulation disorders, we examine their hearing acuity, functions of the speech organs, intelligence and, of course, articulation itself. If we find any need for medical treatment, we advise them to first consult a physician. Speech therapy usually comes after or in cooperation with medical treatment. In the case of cleft palate, for instance, if an operation is successful, speech therapy may not be necessary. The procedure of articulation therapy is roughly divided into two parts: i.e. basic exercise and articulation training.

Basic exercise consists of chewing, sucking and swallowing (CSS) training, and mobility training of the articulatory organs. This is important because the movements of speech organs required in articulation are keenly connected with the movements of speech organs required in eating (as a matter of fact, in speech, we borrow the eating organs).

In the case of articulation disorders with organic defects, CSS training and exercise of speech organs precede the articulation therapy. When the patients have a certain degree of proficiency, they go into articulation training. When there is no organic defect, this training may be omitted.

In articulation training, there are four steps as first suggested by the American speech pathologist, *Charles Van Riper.*

The first step is to establish the auditory image of the correct sound. We give the children correct sound as much as possible and in various situations. The second step is the comparison between the correct sound the others make and the incorrect sound the child makes. If the correct auditory image of a given sound has been established, this step can be finished rather easily. The third step is the production of the correct sound. 'Trial and error' procedures usually take place here. In some cases, we have to use phonetic placement techniques, in which we teach the child the specific place of articulation and the manner of articulation of a given sound.

The fourth step is referred to as 'carry over'. In many cases, it happens that children can pronounce correctly in the training room but not in daily life. We try to carry the correct sound over to their daily lives.

With these steps, we conclude the articulation therapy. Throughout these steps, the auditory aspects are very important, in listening to

Table I. The ratio of speech disorders in school speech classes (%)

	1979 survey (n = 18,810)	1973 survey (n = 12,478)
Articulation	26.5	27.4
Cleft palate	7.0	11.2
Stuttering	13.2	22.9
Hearing	17.6	17.7
Language delay	32.0	20.8
Others	3.7	
Total	100.0	100.0

correct sounds, in comparing correct and incorrect sounds, and of course in producing correct sounds. We always observe the child's capability for auditory discrimination and identification. Fortunately, the prognosis of articulation disorders in children is fairly good. This is because the symbolic function or language performance is intact in most of the cases.

If speech disorders result from language performance, the prognosis is not as good as in the case of articulation disorders. We do not yet even have clear steps for language therapy. However, the ratio of language-delayed children has been increasing. Thus, research on the language therapy technique and related fields should be most important in the future.

Table I and figures 1 and 2 show some statistics on speech therapy for school children. In the result of the 1979 survey, the largest portion is occupied by language delay, and the second by articulation disorders. When we made the same kind of survey in 1973, 6 years earlier, the language-delayed children were less than 20%. 'Early detection and early education' has been the main trend in special education in Japan. So, we take care of preschool children even in school speech classes. The ratio is 28.2% (fig. 2).

In hospital settings, all kinds of speech disorders have been treated for a long time in various fields. For instance, among oto-rhino-laryngologists there have been quite a few doctors who were interested in voice and speech disorders. Many distinguished research works came from this field. Oral surgeons have been interested in cleft palate

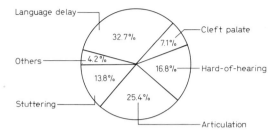

Fig. 1. Speech disorders in schools (n = 21,290).

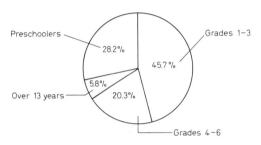

Fig. 2. Ratio by grade (n = 21,290).

speech. Orthopedists have treated cerebral palsy speech. Psychiatrists and physicians have been interested in aphasia and related disorders.

Among them, the leaders have been oto-rhino-laryngologists. They founded the Japan Society of Logopedics and Phoniatrics in the mid-1950s. In the early 1960s, an oto-rhino-laryngological department of a university hospital employed two specialists for speech therapy, and a rehabilitation hospital officially opened a speech clinic. In the field of medicine, however, the increase of the number of therapists and clinics was not so remarkable as in the field of education. We have only one training center which offers a 1-year course to the university graduate. According to the 1979 survey, there are about 600 speech therapists including the graduates of the training center, although qualification for license has not been issued.

I would like to discuss two kinds of speech disorders resulting from cerebral vascular accidents, i.e. aphasia and dysarthria. Aphasia is a disturbance of language performance. The symptoms are quite different according to the type, e.g. motor or sensory aphasia. Some of the symptoms which can be recognized most frequently are 'naming difficulty', 'paraphasia', 'circumlocution', 'perseveration', and 'difficulties in writing and reading'. Language performance includes not only speech but writing and reading, auditory comprehension, and related areas such as calculation and color concept. Most aphasic patients have disorders in all these modalities. Most aphasic patients have paralyzed extremities, usually on the right-hand side, this means that most have to adjust to using the nondominant hand in activities of daily life, and also have to practice walking. Some of them have seizures from time to time. And, as a general effect of brain damage, many aphasics do not have a positive motivation for doing things.

By this brief description of aphasics, one can well imagine that speech therapy for aphasics should be done in a keen team approach. On the basis of this team approach, when we meet an aphasic patient, we evaluate the residual ability in each modality of language. We also try to find out the best combination in reception and expression for each patient. For instance, if there an aphasic patient understands letters better than oral speech, and can express himself better by pointing at pictures or letters, then we ask the people around him to use letters and pictures when communicating with him. Meanwhile, we try to improve his ability to comprehend and express in other modalities. Some aphasic patients can express their ideas if we ask them questions which can be answered by 'yes' or 'no', then we ask the people around them to use that method of communication, even though it is time-consuming.

For any person, the most basic and most effective communicative means is auditory comprehension and oral speech. Most of the patients themselves and their families want to use speech as a matter of naturalness and effectiveness. But they just cannot. Therefore, our first job is to inform them about aphasia and let them use the most suitable mode of communication, at least for the time being. We know that if one modality improves, others also will.

Many patients leave the hospital during the course of therapy. It is interesting to note, however, that even after the termination of speech therapy in the hospital, the patient's ability to communicate keeps improving if the surrounding people are understanding in communicating with him and try to give him mental stability.

The telephone can be used to continue the therapy. The patient calls the hospital at the appointed time and receives oral speech training. This method was first utilized for those patients that lived too far away to visit the hospital as out-patients. To have speech therapy once

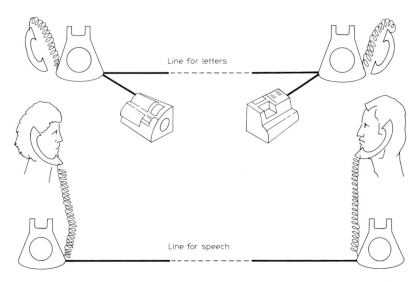

Line for letters

Line for speech

Fig. 3. Telephone therapy at Kanto Teishin Hospital.

a week or even once a month on the phone motivates the patient and gives him a feeling of security.

A recent method is giving the patient writing and reading practice by using an electronic device called telephonephax (fig. 3). In this method, we use two telephone lines, one for oral speech and the other for written material which is sent from or to the patient. It takes 5 min for the copies to arrive, so we could plan another method. Just recently, telephone facsimile has been on the market. By this method we can send written material in real time. We are planning to use this device, too, though it will take a little time for these devices to become popular because of their high cost.

Frankly speaking, restoration of language performance is not as striking as we wish. Most of the patients cannot communicate without various degrees of help from others. The data show that only about 20% of the aphasic patients have returned to their jobs. We try to make the patients and their families understand that complete recovery from aphasia is but a dream although improvement will come slowly and gradually. We try to make this fact understood during the course of training.

The therapeutic principle is the same for dysarthric patients as that mentioned for articulation disorders, because dysarthria is basically a disorder of oral speech, with intact language performance. However, for some severe dysarthric patients, it is quite difficult to improve speaking ability. The patient knows what he wants to say, he chooses the correct words and pronounces them with great effort, but the listener cannot understand them. Every dysarthric patient has the same experiences.

To compensate a little for the problem, a device called a 'communicator' has been developed. It is a portable device, weighing a little over 300 g and measuring about 20×9 cm and has 50 keys of the Japanese alphabet and a printed paper-tape output. By using this device, the time needed for communication is greatly decreased. But the effectiveness of the device depends on the patients' intelligence and motivation. There are some drawback, among them is the listner's reaction, which is astonishment and sometimes resentment because of the strange and troublesome way of communication. These reactions result in reducing patient motivation.

As far as speech intelligibility is concerned, there are many possible ways of compensation. The most important thing to be remembered, however, is that our communication is established by at least two people. We are apt to think that *they are* handicapped, and *we are not*. But, in communication, both speaker and listener are handicapped. We must recognize this fact and have to change our reaction towards them and our way of talking. I think this is more important than the mere cry for an increase in the number of therapists.

1981 was the International Year of Disabled Persons. The number of disabled persons including the communicatively disabled will increase in the future. For the future in Japan, if everybody can share jobs with the disabled and communicate with them, with or without oral speech, and if everybody can share happy times with them, I would say that speech rehabilitation in Japan will be successful. I, as a speech pathologist and an individual, will try to make this dream come true.

T. Nagasawa, D. H. Sc., The National Institute of Special Education, 2360, Nobi, Yokosuka, Kanagawa 239 Pref. (Japan)

Adv. Oto-Rhino-Laryng., vol. 29, pp. 216–223 (Karger, Basel 1983)

Cholesteatoma Surgery; Transcanal Approach

N. Shah

Royal National Throat, Nose and Ear Hospital, London, England

'As to diseases, make a habit of two things; to help or at least do no harm.'

Hippocrates

The first description of cholesteatoma was given by *Cruveilhier* [1] in 1829 and referred to it as a *'pearly tumour'*. The term *cholesteatoma* was given by *Virchow* [2], who described it in greater detail in 1854. The characteristic feature of a cholesteatoma is the presence of keratinizing stratified squamous epithelium within the middle ear cleft. Arguments about the aetiology and its presence in the middle ear cleft will continue, but it is generally accepted that a cholesteatoma sac filled with matrix is a potentially dangerous disease.

The aim of the therapy is to eradicate the disease, preserve or restore cochlear function and prevent recurrence or complication. In some cases this can be achieved by local treatment, but the majority require a radical operation. The surgical procedures practiced are as follows: suction clearance *(Mcgkin)*; atticotomy *(Tumarkin)*; modified radical mastoidectomy *(Bondy)*; radical mastoidectomy *(Zaufal)*; intact canal wall mastoidectomy *(Jansen)*; epitympanotomy with osteoplastic flap *(Wullestein)*. These operations are historical landmarks in mastoid surgery. The simple cortical mastoidectomy [3] to drain mastoid abscess was the most frequently performed operation before the advent of antibiotics. It was established as a life-saving measure, few surgical procedures equalled and none surpassed. However, it was soon recognized that this simple operation failed to cure the cases of cholesteatoma in the attic and in 1890 *Zaufal* [4] described the technique of radical mastoidectomy. This operation converted the attic, antrum, mastoid, tympanum and the external auditory meatus into a common open cavity. It was a generally accepted procedure, but the hearing results were poor.

In order to preserve hearing, *Bondy* [5] in 1910 described a modification to the radical operation in which only part of the posterior and superior bony canal wall was removed, without disturbing the intact pars tensa or the ossicles. This procedure did not gain widespread acceptance until *Lempert's* one-stage fenestration in 1938. Many surgeons continued to practice both procedures until the dramatic introduction of *Tympanoplasty* by *Zöllner* [6] and *Wullestein* [7]. Skin grafts were used to repair the defects in the tympanic membrane, a mastoid cavity was also lined with skin in order to promote healing. Although early tympanoplastic results were encouraging, the long-term results were disappointing. Despite excellent surgery some ears continued to discharge without improvement in hearing levels. Aided by magnification, better light, drugs and new equipment, tympanoplastic techniques have gone through major changes.

First, skin pedicles were used, later free grafts, vein, dura and now temporalis fascia is the preferred technique. Plastic prostheses, stainless steel, cartilage and other materials were tried for replacement of the ossicles, but rejected. Homograft ossicles seem to be in favour at the present time, however, renewed attempts to use new materials in the shape of Torp and Porp are frequently made. The desire to attain near normal anatomical and physiological goals led to the combined-approach tympanoplasty – intact canal wall mastoidectomy by *Jansen* [8]. This procedure was embraced by a number of surgeons in other countries *(Sheehy, Smyth);* however, the early enthusiasm has waned. The combined-approach tympanoplasty is still favoured by some surgeons; others have returned to the two-stage operation or open-cavity procedure.

The main disadvantages of classical radical mastoidectomy are a large cavity, poor hearing and persistent discharge in some cases. These points merit further comments in order to appreciate the present technique.

Large cavity: X-ray studies, analysis of case records and operative findings confirm that over 75–80% of ears with chronic ear disease have poorly pneumatized sclerotic mastoids. The traditional teaching and practice of locating the mastoid antrum first, necessitates a wide conical opening of the normal mastoid bone. Since secondary acquired cholesteatoma is usually confined to the attic and very rarely extends beyond the mastoid antrum, the large cavity can be avoided if the procedure of the bone work is reversed, resulting in a very small cavity.

Poor hearing: In the classical radical operation, the absence of the drumhead and exposed round window membrane leads to poor hearing. In the majority of attic cholesteatomas, the ossicular chain is usually intact and the hearing can be preserved or improved by creating a new but shallow mesotympanum-type III tympanoplasty.

Persistent discharge: In a personal series of revision mastoidectomies, it was apparent that many operations were inadequate. 45% had poor aeration due to inadequate meatoplasty caused by poor technique, stenosis and postaural depression. 40% had high facial ridge and 30% had other problems including granulations, recurrence, open Eustachian tube, etc. Dry ears can only be achieved by adequate meatoplasty and sealing the middle ear by a fascial graft.

The aim of the surgical treatment is to eradicate the disease, make the ear safe by producing a clean, dry, odourless, skin-lined small open cavity and to preserve or improve hearing. This goal can be achieved by a postaural transcanal mastoidectomy with fascial graft. The basic steps of the operation are described as follows:

Operation: The usual preoperative checks and investigations including X-rays and hearing tests are performed. The ear is cleaned the day before surgery, and the operation is performed under general anaesthesia. The patient is positioned with the head inclined to the opposite side and the operative field draped. The ear is examined under the microscope and cleaned. The postaural and canal skin is infiltrated with a solution of epinephrine (1:200,000).

Incision: A posterosuperior incision, a few millimetres behind the postaural groove and above the helix is made through the skin. The soft tissues and pinna are detached and pushed forwards. Haemostasis is completed and a small mastoid retractor is positioned in place. Temporalis fascia is then exposed and an adequate piece is removed and prepared dry for later use. A rectangular flap in the periosteum is made and elevated (fig. 1) to expose the mastoid bone. The exposed spine of

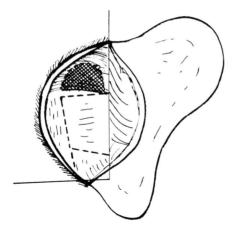

Fig. 1. Posterosuperior incision: temporalis fascia graft and rectangular periosteal flap.

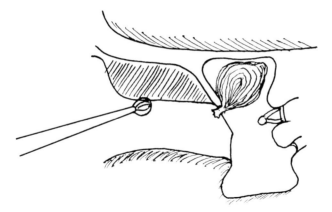

Fig. 2. Bonework: enlarging the bony canal.

Henle is also cleaned and the meatal skin from posterior and superior wall freed, and elevated as a soft tissue pedicle. This may be held out of the field by a retractor or a piece of ribbon gauge.

Bonework: This is performed by a large cutting burr (fig. 2): starting at the spine of Henle, and enlarging the bony canal as far down as the sulcus near the perforation, until the lateral wall of the attic and antrum is almost transparent. The attic is opened through the existing

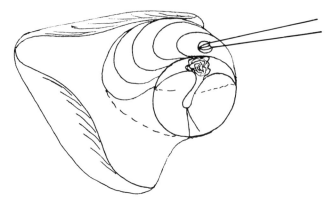

Fig. 3. Bonework: opening the attic, aditus and antrum.

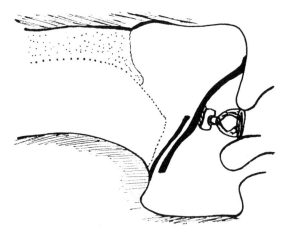

Fig. 4. Shallow middle ear with graft in place: type III tympanoplasty.

perforation by a smaller burr and followed posteriorly and inferiorly to open the aditus and antrum (fig. 3).

Diseased mucous membrane and bone are removed and the status of the ossicular chain is established. It may also be necessary to separate the incudo-stapedial joint at this stage. The cholesteatoma sac with matrix and incus are carefully and completely removed from behind, forwards by suction and elevators. Great care is exercised in the area of the facial nerve and the oval window. Undue suction or mobilization of the stapes superstructure is to be avoided. The malleus is dissected

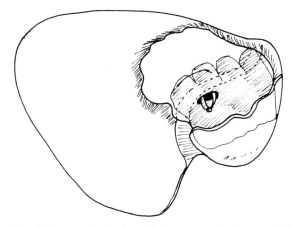

Fig. 5. Temporalis fascia graft in place under the remainder of the tympanic membrane.

free, removed, and the anterior attic space cleaned. The resulting bean-shaped cavity is converted into a round smooth cavity by lowering the facial ridge. In a pneumatized mastoid bone, it may be necessary to create a larger cavity requiring bigger meatoplasty. The dried temporalis fascia graft is then cut to size and placed under the remainder of the drum inferiorly, and over the facial and lateral semicircular canals, creating a shallow, but sealed middle ear. Occasionally a small piece of bone may be placed (fig. 4, 5) over the head of the stapes to make better contact, or a second stage procedure is performed if the stapes superstructure is absent. A silicone disc is then placed over the graft and a small piece of bismuth, iodoform, paraffin paste (BIPP) is inserted to secure the graft.

Meatoplasty: This is perhaps the most important part of the open technique and should be performed with great care. The life-long misery of a smelly, discharging cavity can be avoided by a good meatoplasty. Unfortunately, this is not appreciated by many surgeons. The meatal opening should always be in proportion to the bony cavity [9]. For a small cavity, a small meatoplasty with three flaps – superior, posterior and inferior (fig. 6) may be adequate. In a larger cavity sufficient conchal cartilage must be removed to create opening to allow aeration of the cavity. These skin flaps are secured in place by transfixing sutures. The rectangular periosteal flap is sutured back with the perio-

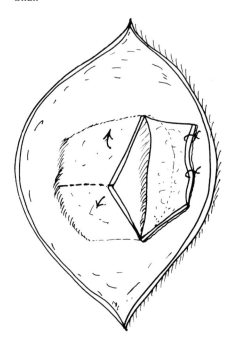

Fig. 6. Meatoplasty flaps.

Table I. Results (1974–1979)

	Cases	
	n	%
Dry ears	67	89
Internal discharge	3	4
Moist cavity	1	1
Wet cavity	4	5

Table II. Hearing results

	Cases	
	n	%
Within 0–15 dB	10	13
Within 15–35 dB	15	20
Within 35–60 dB	35	46
60 dB +	15	20

steum and the wound is closed in layers. An additional BIPP gauge is packed in the cavity and dressings are applied. The mastoid bandage is removed after 24 h and replaced by a light, foam dressing for 5 days. The BIPP pack is removed after 1 week and the cavity is gently cleaned under the microscope. A fresh BIPP is loosely packed and changed at 2-weekly intervals, until the cavity is well epithelialized. Routine oral antibiotics are given for 1 week, and particularly when the cartilage is cut or excised during the meatoplasty.

Results: In a personal series of 75 operations performed during 1974–79, the results for achieving a dry safe ear and hearing level are shown in tables I and II.

References

1   Cruveilhier, L.J.B.: Anatomie pathologique du corpus humani, vol. 1 (Ballière, Paris 1829).
2   Virchow, R.: Über Perlgeschwulste. Virchows Arch. path. Anat. Physiol. *8:* 371 (1854).
3   Schwartze, H.H.; Eysell, C.G.: Über die künstliche Eröffnung des Warzenfortsatzes. Arch. Ohrenheilk. *7:* 157 (1873).
4   Zaufal, E.: Technik der Trepanation des proc. Mastoid nach Kusterschen Grundsätzen. Arch. Ohrenheilk. *30:* 291 (1890).
5   Bondy, G.: Totalaufmeisselung mit Erhaltung von Trommelfell und Gehörknöchelchen. Mschr. Ohrenheilk. *44:* 15 (1910).
6   Zöllner, F.: Die Radikaloperation mit besonderem Bezug auf die Hörfunktion. Z. Lar. Rhinol. Otol. *30:* 104 (1951).
7   Wullestein, H.: Funktionelle Operationen im Mittelohr mit Hilfe des freien Spaltlappen-Transplantates. Arch. Ohr.-Nas.-Kehlk. Heilk. *161:* 422 (1952).
8   Jansen, C.: Über Radikaloperation und Tympanoplastik. Sitz. Ber. Fortbild, Arztek., OBV (1958).
9   Portmann, M.: 'Open' or 'closed' technique in surgery of the middle ear. Ann. Otol. Rhinol. Lar. *77:* 927 (1968).

N. Shah, MD, Royal National Throat, Nose and Ear Hospital,
330/332, Gray's Inn Road, London WC1X 8DA (England)

Adv. Oto-Rhino-Laryng., vol. 29, pp. 224–230 (Karger, Basel 1983)

Zygomycosis in Otorhinolaryngological Practice

F. D. Martinson

Department of Otorhinolaryngology, College of Medicine, University of Ibadan, Ibadan, Nigeria

Zygomycetes is one of the six classes into which the large class Phycomycetes has been subdivided (fig. 1). These ubiquitous fungi are found, as laboratory contaminants, in the soil, on decaying vegetation, in insects and reptiles as well as on human skin and in the upper respiratory tract among other sites. Although they are commonly saprobic or saprophytic, they may under various circumstances become pathogenic to their hosts. The first accepted report of deep infection by the Zygomycetes have been credited to *Cohnheim* [4] and *Fürbringer* [6]. The fungi responsible were of the order Mucorales. Since then these infections collectively called Mucormycoses have attracted the interest of almost every clinical discipline. It is only within the last 30 years, however, that human infections by fungi of the order Entomophthorales have been recognized and reported. These have appropriately been called Entomophthoromycoses [3].

The *Mucormycoses* are usually described as 'opportunistic infections' or more recently by *Vanbreuseghem* [15] and *Vanbreuseghem and Larsh* [16] as 'asthenomycoses'. Both terms imply that the infections occur almost exclusively in the patient whose resistance has been severely compromised either by debilitating illnesses such as diabetes, kwashiorkor, some malignancies and severe gastroenteritis, or by prolonged use of cytotoxic drugs, steroids and immunosuppressives. The infection occurs at all ages and in both sexes and spares no structure or organ. That in the nose – commonly called rhinomucormycosis or rhinocerebral mucormycosis – commences as an ulcerating granuloma in the nasal cavity or paranasal sinuses and spreads outwards to the surface or deeply to the pharynx, the orbit and cranial cavity where meningitis,

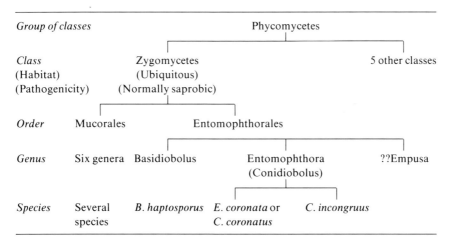

Fig. 1. Zygomycetes in otolaryngological pratice

cerebral haemorrhage, infarcts or abscesses may be terminal complications. Areas of facial pain or of anaesthesia are commonly complained of. Because of the very marked tendency of the fungus to penetrate blood vessels, vascular thromboses and widespread dissemination are common. The clinical picture thus simulates a rapidly advancing malignant tumour with superimposed pyogenic infection.

On histology the lesion consists of inflammatory granulation tissue with neutrophils, few lymphocytes and plasma cells, eosinophils and scanty if any fibroblasts. Hyphae are seen, some penetrating or lying within blood vessels causing thromboses and infarcts.

Treatment is with amphotericin B, but this will succeed only if the underlying precipitating factor is cured, controlled or eliminated as the case may be, assuming complications are not beyond cure. Very few cases with intracranial spread for instance have been known to recover.

The first cases of Entomophthoromycosis were reported by *Joe* et al. [8]. The infection involved the limbs and trunk of Indonesian children, starting and spreading as a granuloma in the subcutaneous fatty tissue. The author [8] therefore called it 'subcutaneous phycomycosis'; but as experience has shown that the granuloma does infiltrate muscle as well, *Vanbreuseghem* [15] renamed it 'basidiobolomycosis' after Basidiobolus, the genus responsible. The infection was soon recognized in tropical Africa and other tropical countries. It occurs, but very rarely, in the temperate climates unlike mucormycosis which is universal. The granuloma is not restricted to the limbs and trunk but does involve, and may start in the neck or face, the field of the otolaryngologist.

Human nasal entomophthoromycosis began to appear or to be recognized about the same time [1, 9]. *Emmons and Bridges* [5] identified the causative organism in similar lesions of horses as *Entomophthora coronata,* and with *Bras* et al. [2] first showed that the causative organism in human nasal infection was also *E. coronata.* This was subsequently confirmed in reports from various parts of the world and the infection acquired the descriptive name 'rhinophycomycosis entomophthorae' [12] and 'rhinoentomophthoromycosis' [3].

The *Entomophthoromycoses* are acquired by implantation of the fungus by an insect or a scratch from a contaminated bit of vegetation or a fingernail. Yet in spite of the widespread distribution of the fungus in nature and the numerous known incidents of such minor trauma, the infection is surprisingly uncommon. As, so far, no recognizable precipitating factor has been discovered, one may speculate that one of the possible reasons for rarity of the infection may be that the pathogenicity of the fungus depends on its state of form in nature at the time of implantation. *Clark* [3] suggested that as there are variations within the species, only a few of these variations may actually be pathogenic to man. She also suggests that as the disease has been known to be self-limiting, some infections may have resolved spontaneously before they could become clinically obvious or significant. It is also possible, I feel, that a degree of immunity is acquired from frequent minimal exposures to the fungus.

Basidiobolomycosis affects principally children and adolescents. It presents as a firm smooth or lobulated mass, movable over deeper tissues and, characteristically, has well-defined palpable edges. It often reaches enormous proportions and extends across anatomical regional boundaries. It is painless, not tender and does not ulcerate unless traumatized. There is no evidence of lymph gland involvement, except as reactive hyperplasia, and no constitutional disturbance due to the infection itself. It does infiltrate muscle sometimes very extensively; this important fact was exemplified in a case involving the neck which ended in death from respiratory obstruction. Aggressive lesions involving the trunk very occasionally spread through a perineal orifice into the pelvis obstructing the ureter and lower bowel. Though this tendency to enter natural orifices has not definitely been reported in the head, in one case, facial basidiobolomycosis was strongly suspected to have spread into the nasal cavity.

Rhinoentomophthoromycosis, the nasal infection in this group commences in the region of the inferior turbinate, the most easily accessible structure to airborne spores and to other modes of infection mentioned earlier. The granuloma spreads submucosally in any direction, e.g. towards the pharynx where it may simulate a benign neoplasm, through ostia and suture lines into paranasal sinuses, on to the dorsum and glabella, to the forehead, eyelids, cheek and upper lip. It usually limits itself to the central part of the face above the level of the angle of the mouth unless traumatized, e.g. by biopsy at the limits of this area, when it may spread beyond it into the parotid and temporal regions. Apart from this the infection has the same physical characteristics as those of basidiobolomycosis except the size attainable, yet facial deformities though much smaller can sometimes be hideous.

Biopsies are best taken from the growing edges where viable fungus can usually be obtained for mycological culture and diagnosis. In the central older areas fibrosis predominates and the fungi found are dying or effete. It is desirable in rhinoentomophthoromycosis to avoid a facial scar; biopsies are therefore ideally taken from the inferior turbinate, but if necessary from the deep surface of the lip (away from the angle) or from the cheek via the buccal sulcus.

Histopathology: Briefly this consists of a chronic inflammatory granuloma with polymorphs, numerous eosinophils, some plasma cells and lymphocytes, foreign body type giant cells, some containing hyphal elements, also varying amounts of fibroblasts, most numerous in older parts of the granuloma. Few microabscesses containing hyphal elements are seen. On HE staining some hyphae are seen surrounded by a granular eosinophilic halo or sleeve described as the Splendore-Hoeppli reaction and considered to be an antigen antibody reaction [18]. Some of the features which differentiate these lesions from mucormycosis are the absence of thrombosis and of hyphae in the blood vessels though they may rarely be seen attempting to penetrate their walls.

Treatment: The early treatment of entomophthoromycosis was with potassium iodide. As much as 2–3 g were given t.d.s. to adults the duration of treatment often had to be prolonged and few cases seemed resistant. Septrin (Burroughs Wellcome) has replaced potassium iodide and has proved more effective in nasal cases [10, 11]. Successful results have also been achieved in basidiobolomycosis. For nasal lesions growing more rapidly than usual, prednisolone, though contraindicated in mucormycosis, is given at the start of treatment and rapidly tailed off. This regimen has proved successful in all of the 17 cases of rhino-entomophthoromycosis treated in the last 11 years and there have been no recurrences. Amphotericin B has not been effective in either of these two infections.

Surgical excision has been avoided in Rhinoentomophthoromycosis, since to date even the most severe cases seen in Nigeria have eventually responded satisfactorily to medication. Neglected cases or those inadequately treated from the start may tax to the limit one's patience and faith in medical treatment and in desperation a surgically scarred face may be preferred to the severe facial deformity caused by the granulomatous masses.

The differential diagnosis of rhinoentomophthoromycosis include nasal polyps, hypertrophic rhinitis, rhinoscleroma, nasal or pharyngeal neoplasm, while lesions which spread on to the face may resemble tubercular leprosy, fibrous dysplasias, dental cyst or goundou. Facial and cervical basidiobolomycosis have the unmistakable features of the infection elsewhere in the body described earlier.

A third member of the family Entomophthorales has been responsible for pulmonary and mediastinal infection in a 3-year-old child in America [7]. It was thought to have followed inhalation of an insect. Symptoms and signs suggested progressive cardiac and pulmonary embarrassment. Diagnosis was made after biopsy through a thoracotomy and the causative organism was found to be *C. incongruus*. The child recovered completely in 3 months on treatment with amphotericin B. This case is mentioned for completeness though it is outside the field of otolaryngology. Since only one case has so far been reported one cannot say if this fungus has a predilection for the lower respiratory tract alone or might in future appear higher up. One might mention also the case of *Ridley and Wise* [13] in which a lesion below the eye spread to the ethmoids and disseminated widely into the cranial, thoracic and abdominal cavities as would severe mucormycoses. The organism isolated, however, resembled the Entomophthorales histologically and mycologically and was considered to be most likely Empusa, a member of this family pathogenic to certain flies. If confirmed this would be the fourth recognized human entomophthoromycosis in the otolaryngologic field.

Following this description of the recognized clinical features of the zygomycoses in otolaryngology one must refer to some reports in the literature which describe gross deviations from the usual observations regarding pathology and clinical features. Thus, in a report of a case with recognized predisposing debilities, an ulcerating spreading necrotizing palatal lesion progressed and ended as one would have expected of a fulminating mucormycotic infection, yet the fungus isolated was reported as *B. haptosporus*. In another in which the lesion described did not really resemble any of the recognized zygomycoses, the fungus isolated was said to be a species of the Entomophthorales. Could these be unusual variations, new mycoses, or double infections? *Symmers* [14] observed that histological demonstration of a fungus in a lesion does not preclude the presence of one or more other diseases at the same site. With advances in modern therapy new modalities may prove successful in the purposes for which they are employed, but may at the same time create opportunism for other and perhaps new diseases. Thorough investigation of any associated diseases and alertness in observation, backed by the full cooperation of a competent mycologist may help to reveal new or unsuspected mycoses. They could also meanwhile obviate errors in diagnoses and, more important still, avoid tragic results in the management of what might otherwise have been treatable cases.

References

1   Ash, J.E.; Raum, M.: An atlas of otolaryngologic pathology, p. 179 (Armed Forces Institute of Pathology, Washington 1956).
2   Bras, G.; Gordon, C.C.; Emmons, C.W.; Prendegast, K.M.; Sugar, M.: A case of Phycomycosis observed in Jamaica: Infection with Entomophthora coronata. Am. J. trop. Med. Hyg. *14:* 141–145 (1965).
3   Clark, B.M.: Epidemiology of phycomycosis; in Wolstenholme, Porter, Systemic mycoses, pp. 179–192 (Churchill, London 1968).
4   Cohnheim: Zwei Fälle von Mycosis der Lungen. Virchows Arch. path. Anat. *33:* 257–260 (1865).
5   Emmons, C.W.; Bridges, C.H.: Entomophthora coronata, the etiologic agent of phycomycosis in horses. Mycologia *53:* 307–312 (1961).
6   Fürbringer, P.: Beobachtungen über Lungenmycose beim Menschen. Virchows Arch. path. Anat. *66:* 330–365 (1876).

7   Gilbert, E.F.; Khoury, G.H.; Pore, R.S.: Histopathological identification of Ento-
    mophthora phycomycosis. Infection in an infant. Archs Path. *90:* 583–587 (1970).
8   Joe, L.K.; Eng, N.I.T.; Pohan, A.; Meulen, H. van der; Emmons, C.W.: Basidiobo-
    lus ranarum as a cause of subcutaneous mycosis in Indonesia. Archs. Derm.
    74: 378–383 (1956).
9   Martinson, F.D.: Rhinophycomycosis. J. Lar. Otol. *77:* 691–705 (1963).
10 Martinson, F.D.: Chronic phycomycosis of the upper respiratory tract. Phycomyco-
    sis entomophthorae. Am. J. trop Med. Hyg. *20:* 449–455 (1971).
11 Martinson, F.D.: Upper respiratory infection due to Conidiobolus coronatus.
    'Rhinoentomophthoromycosis'; in Takahashi, ISIAN: International Symposium
    of Infections and Allergy of the Nose and Paranasal Sinuses, pp. 170–174
    (SCIMED Publ. Inc., Tokyo 1976).
12 Martinson, F.D.; Clark, B.M.: Rhinophycomycosis entomophthorae in Nigeria.
    Am. J. Med. Hyg. *16:* 40–47 (1967).
13 Ridley, D.S.; Wise, M.J.: Unusual disseminated infection with a phycomycete. J.
    Path. Bact. *90:* 675–679 (1965).
14 Symmers, W.S.C.: Aspects of contribution of histopathology to the study of deep-
    seated fungal infections; in Wolstenholme, Porter, Systemic mycoses (Churchill,
    London 1968).
15 Vanbreuseghem, R.: Guide pratique de mycologie médical et vétérinaire (Masson,
    Paris 1966).
16 Vanbreuseghem, R.; Larsh, H.W.: Conclusions to the round table on the global
    problems due to opportunistic fungi; in Iwati, Recent advances in medical and ve-
    terinary mycology, p. 253 (University of Tokyo Press, Tokyo 1977).
17 Vanbreuseghem, R.; Vroey, C. De: Systemic opportunistic fungal infections. Post-
    grad. med. J. *55:* 593–594 (1979).
18 Williams, A.O.; Lichtenberg, F. von; Smith, J.H.; Martinson, F.D.: Ultrastructure
    of phycomycosis due to Entomophthora, Basidiobolus and associated Splendore
    Hoeppli phenomenon. Archs. Path. *87:* 459–468 (1969).

F. D. Martinson, MD, Department of Otolaryngology, College of Medicine,
University of Ibadan, Ibadan (Nigeria)

Adv. Oto-Rhino-Laryng., vol. 29, pp. 231–234 (Karger, Basel 1983)

Free Papers

Ear

1   Preservation of Tympanic Homografts in Honey: Kailash Rai, Mahendra K. Nuwal, Nilima Duggal (Department of Otolaryngology, Ravindra Nath Takore Medical College, Udaipur, Raj., India)
2   Mycoplasma Otitis – An Outbreak at Kamput Holding Center for Kampuchean Refugees, Chanthaburi Province, Thailand: Amporn Sukonthaman, John D. Freeman, Mai Ratanavararak (Department of Laboratory Medicine, Faculty of Medicine, Chulalongkorn University, Bangkok, Thailand)
3   Aural Histoplasmosis: Primary Cutaneous with Disseminated Histoplasmosis, A Case report: Chalee Kanchanarak, Kobkiat Ruckphaopunt (Department of Otolaryngology, Faculty of Medicine, Chieng Mai University, Chiengmai, Thailand)
4   Some Experiences with Tympanoplasty on Otitis Media Chronica with Cholesteatoma, Preliminary Report: Zainul A. Djaafar (ENT Department, University of Indonesia, Medical School Ciptomangunkusumo Hospital, Jakarta, Indonesia)
5   Tympanoplasty as An Office Procedure: Buddy Y.K. Wong (Kowloon, Hong Kong)
6   Otosclerosis in Thailand: Prasit Srisomboon (Department of Otolaryngology, Faculty of Medicine and Siriraj Hospital, Mahidol University, Bangkok, Thailand)
7   Impedance Audiometry with Otological Diagnosis: Nualnipha Phanijphand (Poplar Bluff Ear, Nose and Throat Clinic, Missouri, USA)
8   Studies on the Round Window Membrane: Akikazu Ito, Hiromu Miyake (Department School of Medicine, Nagoya, Japan)
9   Labyrinthine Window Ruptures: A.D. Cheesman (The Royal National Throat, Nose and Ear Hospital, London, England)
10 The Otolaryngological and Audiological Evaluation in the Traffic Policemen in Bangkok: Sunanta Polpathapee, Somsi Chiwapong (Audiology and Speech Unit, Department of Otolaryngology, Faculty of Medicine and Siriraj Hospital, Mahidol University, Bangkok, Thailand)
11 A Mild Acute Head Injury, Correlation Between Central Hearing Disorders and EEG Changes: P. Tuohimaa, A. Salmivalli, J. Partanen (ENT Clinic, University Central Hospital of Turku, Finland)
12 Tinnitus in Thailand: Suchitra Prasansuk, Ronald Hinchcliffe (Department of Otolaryngology, Faculty of Medicine and Siriraj Hospital, Mahidol University, Bangkok, Thailand)
13 Vestibular Neurectomy in Intractable Vertigo: Carlos P. Reyes (Capitol Medical Center, Manila, Philippines)

Nose

1 Sinoscopy of the Maxillary Sinus at Siriraj Hospital, A Preliminary Report: Vathana Thitadilok, Chern Sekorarithi (Department of Otolaryngology, Faculty of Medicine and Siriraj Hospital, Bangkok, Thailand)

2 Nasopharyngeal Carcinoma: C. Das (Department of Otolaryngology, Silchar Medical College, Silchar Assam, India)

3 Lateral Rhinotomy: Nusjirwan Rifki, Soerjadi Kartosoediro (ENT Department, Faculty of Medicine, University of Indonesia, Jakarta, Indonesia)

4 Nasopharyngeal Angiofibroma, A Rational Treatment Approach: Abhaya Prathap Singh (Department of Otorhinolaryngology, Faculty of Medicine, University of Malaya, Kuala Lumpur, Malaysia)

5 Extensions of Juvenile Nasopharyngeal Angiofibromas into Neighbouring Structures: Purnaman S. Pandi (ENT Department, Faculty of Medicine, University of Indonesia, Jakarta, Indonesia)

6 Juvenile Nasopharyngeal Angiofibroma (JNA), Radiological Aspects: Priya Khanjanasthiti, Wiyda Bhoopat, Chern Sekorarithi, Suthisak Suthipongchai (Department of Radiology, Faculty of Medicine and Siriraj Hospital, Bangkok, Thailand)

7 Preoperative Embolization and Surgery of Juvenile Angiofibroma of the Nasopharynx: Chern Sekorarith, Wiyada Bhoopat (Department of Otolaryngology, Faculty of Medicine and Siriraj Hospital, Mahidol University, Bangkok, Thailand)

8 Xylocaine (10%) and 2 Cases of Leech in Nasal Cavity (1976–1977): Krishnachai Chaiporn (Surgical Division, Vajira Hospital, Bangkok, Thailand)

9 Chemical Ablation of Rhinoscleroma: Kailash Rai (Department of Otolaryngology, Ravindra Nath Takore Medical College, Udaipur, Raj., India)

10 Olfactory Neuroblastoma: Averdi Roezin, A.N. Kurniawan (ENT Department, University of Indonesia, Jakarta, Indonesia)

11 Radiological Evaluation of the Inferior Orbital Fissure: Kiichi Haruyama, Schozo Kawamura, Haruhisa Horikawa (Department of Otorhinolaryngology, Juntendo University, School of Medicine, Tokyo, Japan)

12 The Significance of Aeroallergens in Allergic Rhinitis Patients in Cholburi, Thailand: Narongsak O. Chareon, Boonchua Dhorranintra, Supatra Limpanon (ENT Department, Cholburi Hospital, Cholburi, Thailand)

13 Serum Immunoglobulin E Level in Healthy and Some Allergic Thai Patients: Boonchua Dhorranintra, Chaweewan Bunnag (Department of Pharmacology, Faculty of Medicine and Siriraj Hospital, Mahidol University, Bangkok, Thailand)

14 The Significance of Allergy as An Etiologic Factor in Nasal Polyps: Chaweewan Bunnag, Prasert Pacharee, Prasert Vipulakom, Chana Siriyananda (Department of Otolaryngology, Faculty of Medicine and Siriraj Hospital, Bangkok, Thailand)

15 Nasal Glial Heterotopia: Soejipto Damayanti, Darnila Fachruddin, A.N. Kurniawan (ENT Department, Faculty of Medicine, University of Indonesia, Jakarta, Indonesia)

16 Craniofacial Resection of Ethmoidal Tumours: A.D. Cheesman (The Royal National Throat, Nose and Ear Hospital, London, England)

Throat

L. Tobing (ENT Department, Faculty of Medicine, University of North Sumatra, Medan, Indonesia)

17 Puncture Treatment with Newly Designed Needle for Peritonsillar Abscess: Hajime Aramaki, Haruko Aizawa, Takehisa Fujishiro, Yoko Umeda (Department of Otorhinolaryngology, Tokyo Women's Medical College, Tokyo, Japan)

18 Malignant Lymphoma of the Tonsil: A.N. Kurniawan and A. Harryanto R (Department of Anatomic Pathology, Faculty of Medicine, University of Indonesia, Jakarta, Indonesia)

19 The Use of New Laryngeal Anesthetic Tube for Microlaryngeal Surgery: Thara Tree-Trakan, Apichai Vitavasiri (Department of Anesthesiology and Otolaryngology, Faculty of Medicine, Siriraj Hospital, Mahidol University, Bangkok, Thailand)

Others

1 Embolisation in ENT: N. Kunaratnam (Ear, Nose and Throat Department, Singapore General Hospital, Singapore)

2 Free Rural E.N.T. Project: Salyaveth Lekagul, Soontorn Antarasena, Navarat Thongthai (In private practice, Bangkok, Thailand)

3 Head and Neck Infection Related to Upper Airway Obstruction: Suwan Phanijphand (Poplar Bluff Ear, Nose and Throat Clinic, Missouri, USA)

4 Experiences with CO_2 Laser Surgery: N. Kunaratnam (Ear, Nose and Throat Department, Singapore General Hospital, Singapore)